RAND

An Implicit Review Method for Measuring the Quality of In-hospital Nursing Care of Elderly Congestive Heart Failure Patients

Marjorie L. Pearson, Betty Chang, Jan Lee, Katherine L. Kahn, Lisa V. Rubenstein

Supported by the
National Institute of Nursing Research

PREFACE

In October 1993, researchers at RAND, the UCLA School of Nursing, and the Center for the Study of Healthcare Provider Behavior at the Sepulveda VA Medical Center began a study, funded by the National Institute of Nursing Research, to measure and analyze the quality of nursing care. The objectives of this four-year project are 1) to develop and implement an implicit review method for measuring the quality of nursing care delivered to acutely ill, hospitalized Medicare patients, 2) to evaluate the reliability and validity of this method, including the link between the quality of the process of nursing care and outcomes of care, and 3) to compare the results of this implicit review of nursing care with previously-obtained results of explicit review of nursing care and implicit and explicit review of physician care.

Two diseases were selected for study: congestive heart failure and cerebrovascular accident. While the method for assessing the quality of the nursing care to patients with both diseases is the same, the instruments differ to take account of nursing processes and patient problems particular to one disease. This RAND MR documents the development of the nursing implicit review method and includes the Implicit Review Form and Instruction Manual for reviewing nursing care to congestive heart failure patients. For the Cerebrovascular Accident Implicit Review Form and Instruction Manual, see:

> Marjorie L. Pearson, Betty Chang, Jan Lee, Katherine L. Kahn, and Lisa V. Rubenstein, *An Implicit Review Method for Measuring the Quality of In-hospital Care of Elderly Cerebrovascular Accident Patients*, RAND MR-784-NINR, 1997.

The evaluation of the implicit review methods for CHF and CVA and the comparison of the results of implicit and explicit review methods will be reported separately upon completion.

The research team combines expertise in the fields of nursing, medicine, health policy, quality of care, and study methods, including both implicit and explicit review methodology. The team includes:

- Marjorie L. Pearson, PhD, MSHS, Policy Analyst in the Health Sciences Program at RAND, Santa Monica, California.

- Betty Chang, DNSc, RN, FNP, FAAN, Professor in the School of Nursing at the University of California, Los Angeles.

- Jan Lee, PhD, RN, CS, Associate Professor and Director of Undergraduate and Non-Traditional Programs in the University of Michigan School of Nursing.

- Katherine L. Kahn, MD, Senior Natural Scientist at RAND and practicing internist and Professor of Medicine at the UCLA School of Medicine.

- Lisa V. Rubenstein, MD, MSPH, Senior Natural Scientist at RAND and practicing internist and Associate Clinical Professor of Medicine at the UCLA School of Medicine and Sepulveda VA Medical Center.

CONTENTS

TABLES

SUMMARY

The purpose of this RAND MR is to document the development of an implicit review method for assessing the quality of in-hospital nursing care for congestive heart failure patients. The steps described include the adoption of a conceptual framework for nursing quality, expert nursing panel review, development and pilot testing of the Congestive Heart Failure Implicit Review Form and Instruction Manual, and the selection and training of reviewers. Key principles of implicit review are summarized, and the medical record sample is described. The Congestive Heart Failure Implicit Review Form and the Instruction Manual themselves are included in Appendices B and C.

The Congestive Heart Failure Implicit Review Form consists of 19 questions. To structure the review, these questions guide the reviewer through specific aspects of nursing process: 1) assessment, 2) identification of problems, and 3) problem management, including development of plans, goals, and expected outcomes; nursing interventions; and evaluation of outcomes. After requiring the reviewer to consider each of these aspects of nursing care, the form asks reviewers to rate the overall quality of care. It also asks for information on the patient's nursing needs and acuity, expected outcomes, adverse events, and charting methods.

ACKNOWLEDGMENTS

We gratefully acknowledge the invaluable contribution of the nine nurses who provided detailed review and consultation on our approach to assessing quality of nursing care:

Andee Alsip, M.S.N., C.N.R.N., C.C.M.
San Bernardino, CA

Cora G. Barrios, M.S.N., B.S.N., R.N.
Los Angeles, CA

Zelpha Marie Burbank, M.B.A., B.A., R.N.
Los Angeles, CA

Kathleen Gallagher Epstein, M.N., R.N.
Venice, CA

Lily A. Flores, M.N., R.N.
Glendale, CA

Bonnie L. Jones, M.S.N., R.N., C.N.A.A.
West Covina, CA

Denise Orthen-Armijo, M.S.N., B.S.N., R.N.
Culver City, CA

Lois Ramer, D.N.Sc. F.N.P., R.N.
Whittier, CA

Sandra Elders Rothwell, M.S.N., R.N.
Thousand Oaks, CA

We are equally indebted to the ten nurse reviewers who provided careful review of the 292 congestive heart failure patient records, as well as insightful questions and comments during training. The nurse reviewers included:

Susan J. Bennett, D.N.S., R.N.
Indianapolis, IN

Ginger S. Braun, M.S.N, R.N., C.C.R.N.
Irvine, CA

Clover A. Collins, B.S.N., A.S.N., R.N.C.
Gainesville, FL

Shirley M. Kedrowski Cottingham, M.S.N., R.N.
Palo Alto, CA

Rebecca E. Heffler, M.N., R.N.
Culver City, CA

Esther Kawamura, B.S.N., R.N.
Belmont, CA

Denise Orthen-Armijo, M.S.N., B.S.N., R.N.
Culver City, CA

Molly Sebastian, M.S.N, R.N., C.C.R.N.
Emmaus, PA

Stephanie Tabone, B.S.N., R.N.
Austin, TX

Mary J. Wong, M.S.N., R.N.
San Francisco, CA

We wish to thank Jeri Jackson for providing secretarial support, Carole Oken for assisting with the administrative details of the training, and Alissa Simon and Barbara Simon for assisting with the instrument design.

The study was supported by grant NR03681 issued by the National Institute of Nursing Research. We are grateful for this support.

1. INTRODUCTION

As health care institutions struggle to improve quality while containing costs, quality measurement has become a central focus. Valid and reliable tools are critical for measuring the quality of care delivered by nurses and other key providers. We have developed a method for assessing the quality of nursing care for purposes of internal and external quality review, benchmarking, educational guidance, and nursing research.

Our measure of the process of nursing care uses implicit review of the medical record. The medical record is the most easily accessible and most heavily used source of information on the quality of care received by hospitalized patients. Nurses, in particular, expend considerable resources on charting. Evidence from physician quality review studies supports the notion that the true quality of care received by patients bears a strong relationship to quality of care as recorded in the medical record (Lyons and Payne, 1974). In some studies, patients who receive higher quality of care as judged by medical records have been found to have better outcomes (Rubenstein, Mates, and Sidel, 1977; Kahn, Rogers et al., 1990; Rubenstein, Kahn et al., 1990; Kahn, Draper et al., 1992).

Implicit review of the medical record bases the assessment of quality of care on health care professionals' own judgment; explicit review, in contrast, relies on preset criteria for assessing quality. Implicit review by expert clinicians is the most commonly used gold standard for judging quality, and has the advantage of being more easily applied than explicit review for a variety of diseases and settings (Rubin, Rogers et al., 1992). However, while nurses' notes are generally not excluded from implicit reviews, they have not been the focus of these reviews, nor have nurses been included among the reviewers (Moorehead, Donaldson, and Seravalli, 1971; Richardson, 1972;

Rubenstein, Kahn et al., 1990; Rubenstein, Kahn et al., 1991; Rubin, Kahn et al., 1990).

Nurses carry out complex diagnostic and therapeutic actions during the course of an acute medical hospitalization. Many of these actions are recorded in the nurses' notes section of the medical record. While researchers have focused on reviewing nurses' notes to assess the quality of specific nursing processes, only recently have they begun to focus attention on the link between nursing processes and patient outcomes or the relationship between the quality of nursing care and other dimensions of health care quality, such as the quality of physician care or the appropriate use of services. Currently, there is heightened concern for the identification of nursing sensitive quality measures and methods that facilitate these broader analyses (Rantz, 1995; Lang et al., 1990; Lang and Clinton, 1984; Johnson and Maas, 1994; McCormick, 1991; National Center for Nursing Research, 1992).

We expect that the nursing implicit review method described here will be the foundation for future studies of nursing effectiveness and will be further tested to identify the relationship between care processes and patient outcomes. Nursing research on quality of care thus far has focused almost exclusively on explicit process criteria and on outcome data. Implicit review provides a relatively practical gold standard for everyday use in medical centers for evaluating records that are suspected of demonstrating poor care, or for randomly reviewing records as part of continuous quality improvement efforts.

To develop this implicit review method, we first adopted a conceptual framework for thinking about processes of nursing care. We then designed a form and training and review protocols for implicitly reviewing the medical record to assess nursing quality. Following the lead of the Rubenstein, Kahn et al. (1989; 1991) research in Structured Implicit Review (SIR) of clinician quality, we used our conceptual framework as the basis for studying nursing quality. It guided how we structured the review form and protocols (i.e., the components of nursing quality and data sources specified). In structuring the review, we sought to reduce variation in judgment due to differences in the way the record was reviewed, the data sources, or the components of quality being assessed, while continuing to allow for true differences of opinion on quality.

We are using the implicit review method to assess congestive heart failure (CHF) and cerebrovascular accident (CVA) care. While the method is the same, the instruments reflect some differences in nursing processes for these two categories of patients. This document focuses on the instrument for reviewing the care delivered to CHF patients.

We used a nationally representative sample of medical records of Medicare patients over 65 years admitted to the hospital in 1981-82 and 1984-85 with a primary diagnosis of congestive heart failure. These study records were previously collected and deidentified as part of a national RAND-HCFA quality of care study (Kahn, Rubenstein et al., 1990; Draper et al., 1990; Kahn, Draper et al., 1992). The records were duplicates of complete medical records from 297 hospitals in five states representing different regions of the United States. To maximize the chance of identifying patients for whom death occurred as a result of poor quality, in-hospital deaths were oversampled. Data will be reweighted during the analysis to achieve representativeness of all Medicare patients hospitalized with congestive heart failure.

The use of prior study records has provided the advantage of economically allowing comparison between our nurse implicit review judgments and existing data on the results of physician implicit and explicit review of quality of care. We believe that this advantage outweighs the disadvantage that the records are not current. While our previous research leads us to expect that the fundamental relationships under study are likely to be stable over time (Kahn, Draper, et al., 1992), we plan to evaluate time trend data where appropriate to investigate if nursing process changed over time.

In the following sections, we discuss development of this method of implicit review. Section II describes how we developed the conceptual framework. Section III details the selection and training of the reviewers and the administration of the implicit review of CHF records. In Section IV, we describe the development of the implicit review instrument and instructions. The full text of the Congestive Heart Failure Implicit Review Form and Instruction Manual are included as Appendices B and C.

2. DEVELOPING THE CONCEPTUAL FRAMEWORK

INITIAL STEPS

To develop a structured implicit review form for assessing quality of nursing care, the research team reviewed key literature on nursing theory and practice (Gordon, 1994; Carnevali, 1984). Based on the literature and clinical judgment, we developed a conceptual framework for nursing processes of care. This framework divided nursing care into the following parts:

- assessing and collecting data on the patient,
- defining the problem, and
- managing the problem through
    - setting goals
    - intervening
    - evaluating the success or failure of the intervention.

Our second challenge was to develop a measurement system to evaluate nursing processes of care. Using nursing care literature (Burrell, 1992; Carpenito, 1991; Carpenito, 1993; Thompson, 1993) and the clinical expertise of the research team nurses and physicians, we identified processes of care and quality review criteria critical to each part of the framework for congestive heart failure. By quality review criteria, we mean standards against which the process of care can be evaluated. Thirty-six categories of processes were identified as critical to <u>assessing and collecting data</u> on the patient, and standards for reviewing the adequacy of these processes were specified. For example, assessing allergies was included under initial assessment. The process was to "ask patients about allergies to food or medications" and the standard for reviewing this process was "record presence or absence of allergies at least one time during the first shift." Eleven potential complications of congestive heart failure, e.g., pulmonary edema, were listed as tracer problems that could be considered indicative of the overall quality of <u>problem management</u>. For each tracer problem, processes and standards were specified for developing goals for the problem, intervening, and evaluating the intervention. As an example, CHF patients were defined as being at high risk for pulmonary edema or pulmonary congestion if they had shortness of breath, pulse > 130, respiratory rate > 30, or cyanosis (documented in physician or nursing notes.) One nursing intervention process was to "check breath sounds" and the standard was to "chart breath sounds in medical record within two shifts of onset."

The research team then drafted an implicit review form, using both the conceptual framework and the quality review criteria to structure the form. The review form aimed to encourage similarities in the way the review is approached and in the components of quality being assessed, so that variations in reviewers' judgment reflect true differences of opinion on quality.

EXPERT NURSING PANEL

We next assembled a panel of nine nurse consultants with experience in quality of care assessment to review our approach. To construct a list of potential candidates for this panel, we consulted with an elected representative of a statewide nurses' association and a dean of a school of nursing. Potential candidates received a letter describing the project, inquiring if they were interested in participating, and requesting those interested to provide information on their nursing backgrounds for purposes of balancing the panel. Of 32 potential candidates, 19 expressed interest in participating, of which 9 were selected based on their quality review and nursing experience, as well as their availability. All nine consultants were experienced in quality review and in caring for CHF and CVA patients.

The research team sent the drafts of the conceptual framework, the quality review criteria, and the structured implicit review form, along with relevant definitions and articles pertinent to measuring the quality of nursing care, to the nurse consultants prior to the panel meeting. The nurse consultants were asked to prepare for the meeting by reading the materials and reviewing all of the suggested processes and standards for nursing care of congestive heart failure patients. They were asked to rate the <u>desirability</u> of evaluating each process by indicating whether measuring the process was essential, preferable, acceptable, or not useful. Similarly, they were asked to rate the <u>availability</u> of documentation about each process in the medical record by indicating whether documentation would be available, relatively available, somewhat available, or not available. As an example, Table 1 shows three processes the nurses were asked to rate. At the panel meeting, the nurses discussed and critiqued their ratings of these processes, as well as the conceptual framework and the implicit review form.

Based on the panel discussions, the research team revised the conceptual framework, quality review criteria, and implicit review form. The consultants were sent a revised list of processes and asked to again rate them. They included a similar scale for rating the <u>desirability</u> of evaluating each process as a measure of quality, but, based on a distinction made in the panel discussion, two new rating scales were substituted for the previous scale on availability rating. One asked the panelists to rate the <u>likelihood that the process is performed</u> by good nurses and the other asked them to rate the <u>likelihood that the process is documented</u> in the medical record when it is performed. Standards for reviewing the adequacy of the processes were eliminated from this list for space reasons. Table 2 provides an example of four processes and these rating scales. The information gained from these ratings was taken into account in subsequent revisions of the implicit review form, as well as in the instructions for the review.

PILOT

After revising the implicit review form, the research team drafted detailed instructions for completing the form. The drafts of the form and the instructions were then sent to the consultants. They were asked to review and critique the form, and use it to complete pilot reviews of three CHF medical records. Subsequently, both the form and the instructions were again revised based on the consultants' pilot reviews and comments.

3. PERFORMING IMPLICIT REVIEW

REVIEWER SAMPLE

The project's protocol called for ten implicit reviewers: six from California (to reduce traveling costs) and one from each of the other four states from which the team had medical records (Florida, Indiana, Pennsylvania, and Texas).

Selection Process

After receiving a letter of support from the American Nurses Association, the research team asked the state nurses associations in the five study states to assist in recruiting qualified nurse reviewers with 1) a minimum of a baccalaureate degree in nursing, 2) contact with the day to day care of patients in an acute hospital, 3) some experience in reviewing patient records, e.g., participation in utilization review, and 4) the ability to recognize good nursing care, but at a level achievable by motivated practitioners under average conditions at any average U.S. hospital.

The state nurses' associations were asked to send up to five names, in order of preference. They also were requested to ask the nominees to complete the project's Nursing Background Form (contained in Appendix A) which included questions on the nurse's experience in specified types of care and quality of care assessment. In situations where the state nurses' association failed to produce nominees, the research team requested assistance from schools of nursing or university or community hospitals in those states. This recruitment process yielded 33 candidates.

The research team sent letters of invitation to the candidates who were listed as first preference by the state nurses' associations. The remaining reviewers were selected from among the nurses suggested by schools of nursing or university or community hospitals on the basis of their background characteristics so as to balance the group of reviewers with respect to their experience in types of care, types of hospitals, quality of care assessment, and ethnicity. The first ten invitees all accepted.

Description of Expertise/Background

Tables 3-5 summarize the nursing experience represented by these implicit reviewers. Sizable proportions were experienced in the care of patient populations similar to our sample (geriatric CHF and geriatric CVA patients) and in quality of care assessment.

REVIEWER TRAINING

Training Seminar

The ten reviewers were brought to RAND in Santa Monica for a one-day training seminar on implicit review of medical records. To acquaint them with the implicit review process, project staff mailed them a draft review form and medical record in advance of the training. At the session, they were provided with two binders. One contained the agenda for the day, a listing of the reviewers and the research team, a project summary, the project's conceptual framework for studying the process of nursing care, pertinent definitions (e.g., implicit review of medical records and nursing intervention), and administrative documents (e.g., oath of confidentiality). The second binder contained the draft of the instruction manual and the implicit review form.

Following introductory presentations on the project goals and nursing quality assessment, the reviewers were asked to spend an hour rating a sample medical record using the implicit review form. They then discussed this review in detail with the project research team. For each question on the form, the group went over where they agreed and disagreed in interpreting the question and the rating scale for the sample medical record. The research team answered the reviewers' questions, took note of all inquiries and problems raised by the reviewers, and stressed the key points and how they applied in that case. Following this discussion, the reviewers were asked to review a second medical record and again discuss this review in detail.

Practice Reviews

Immediately after the training seminar, the research team revised the implicit review form and the instruction manual based on the questions and problems experienced during the seminar. The team mailed the revised versions of these documents and three more sample medical records to the reviewers for practice reviews. Three two-hour conference calls were used to discuss each question and achieve consensus in their use of data sources, interpretation of the rating scales, and understanding of the questions and the types of quality being assessed.

Key Principles Emphasized

Throughout the training, the research team emphasized the key principles of implicit review delineated at the beginning of the instruction manual. The following points were frequently reiterated:

- Think about the probable effect of the care given on the patient's chance of a good outcome when judging the quality of nursing care. Out of 100 patients in the same clinical state as the patient under review, how many would have suffered an adverse outcome if treated this way, compared to the number who would have done so if treated optimally?

- Remember that we are interested in whether the patient's needs were met, not in assigning blame, finding reasons for omissions, nor assessing how difficult it was to meet the patient's needs.

- Do not infer actions or events, but, rather, judge solely on the basis of the record.

- Use your recollection of 1980's standards of nursing care for assessing what the patient needed.

- Do not lower your expectations about the assessments and interventions needed by patients with "do not resuscitate" orders.

- Save the highest and lowest ratings for care that is truly excellent or very poor respectively. The highest or lowest rating should mean that you would not want to distinguish any better or worse care.

- Do not be concerned if your judgments vary somewhat from other reviewers. We want to reduce variation due to arbitrary methodological differences, such as those due to different interpretation of the rating scales, but allow for true differences of opinion on what should be done.

REVIEWS

The research team incorporated what they learned during the conference calls into the final revisions of the implicit review form and instruction manual. The team then mailed each reviewer a summary of the conference call training discussions, the final version of the instruction manual, the deidentified medical records of congestive heart failure patients, copies of the implicit review form, and administrative materials.

The medical records were randomly assigned to the reviewers. To separate the variation in quality among states from the variation in assessment among reviewers, each reviewer received medical records from all five states. To measure interrater reliability, a sample of 90 of the 292 records was distributed to two reviewers. Altogether the reviewers each received 38 - 39 records of patients with CHF.

4. CONGESTIVE HEART FAILURE IMPLICIT REVIEW FORM AND INSTRUCTION MANUAL

FORM

Development

As is evident in the previous sections, the structured implicit review form went through numerous revisions. In addition to the multiple changes made in discussions among the project members, the form was reviewed and critiqued by the panel of nurse consultants, piloted and revised, and then revised at different stages throughout the training process.

The project's conceptual framework guided the structure of the implicit review form. The form consists of 19 questions. These questions guide the reviewer through specific aspects of <u>assessment</u> (questions 1 and 7); <u>identification of problems</u> (questions 3 and 5A); and <u>problem management</u>, including development of plans, goals, and expected outcomes (question 5B), nursing interventions (questions 2, 5C, and 6), and evaluation of outcomes (question 5D). After requiring the reviewer to consider each of these aspects of nursing care, the form asks reviewers to rate the overall quality of care (questions 14 - 17). It also asks for information on the patient's nursing needs and acuity (questions 4 and 10 - 12), expected outcomes (question 13), adverse events (questions 8 - 9), and charting methods (questions 7 and 18 - 19). Table 6 classifies the questions by which aspects of care and hospitalization time period are reviewed.

The final version of the Congestive Heart Failure Implicit Review Form can be found in Appendix B.

Allowable Data Sources And Time Periods

For each quality judgment, the data sources and the time period were specified in the review form or instruction manual. The objective was to encourage the reviewers to assign ratings based on the same information in the medical record. A number of questions required the reviewers to first assess what was needed and then to assess the nursing response to these needs; allowable data sources and time were specified for both assessments. For example, to assess nurse implementation of physician orders for vital signs and weight, the reviewers were told to use the physician order sheets for days 1 and 2 of the hospitalization to identify the physicians' orders and to use all relevant sections of the medical record (e.g., TPR records, flowsheets, nurses' notes) for the first 5 days of the patient's hospitalization (or the length of the hospitalization if the stay was shorter than 5 days) to assess the nurses' implementation of these orders.

To rate the nurses' assessment of the patient's needs and health status, the reviewers were told to use the whole medical record to understand the patient's condition and to use only data recorded by nurses (nurse notes, admission and discharge notes, temperature, pulse, and respiration sheets, medication sheets, flowsheets, and specific data sheets, e.g., patient education and skin care) to judge the quality of the nurse assessment. Specific time periods were attached to each kind of assessment. Reviewers were to examine data recorded for days 1 and 2 of the hospitalization to judge the initial assessment; data for days 3 through 10 of the hospitalization or through 1 day prior to discharge, whichever came first, for the reassessment; and data for the day of and day prior to discharge for the pre-discharge assessment.

For the questions asking for summary quality judgments, the reviewers were allowed to use all relevant data in the parts of the medical record and the time periods already reviewed for the other questions.

Table 6 shows the period of hospitalization covered by each question.

INSTRUCTION MANUAL

The instruction manual was drafted to provide more guidance to the question by question rating than could be provided on the form. Following the guideline format previously used in the implicit review of the quality of physician care (Kahn, Rubenstein et al., 1989), the manual described the purpose, data sources, rating scale, and, where appropriate, the specific items for each question on the implicit review form.

The instruction manual also went through multiple revisions with particularly close attention paid to problems suggested during the course of the reviewer training. The text of the Congestive Heart Failure Instruction Manual is presented in Appendix C.

TABLE 1

ASSESS/SEARCH FOR PROBLEMS

I. Initial Assessment (Day 1 or Day 2) Generating Nursing Data Base

A. General Health Status Assessment

	RATING SCALES	
	Rate the Desirability of Evaluating Each Process 3 – Essential 2 – Preferable 1 – Acceptable 0 – Not useful	Rate the Availability of Documentation About Process in the Medical Record 3 – Available 2 – Relatively available 1 – Somewhat available 0 – Not available
PROCESS:	Desirability of evaluating process. (Circle one)	Availability of process in record (Circle one)

Assessment 1. Vital signs

Measure:
- Temperature
- Pulse
- Respiration rate
- Blood pressure

STANDARD: Record during the shift patient is admitted

Desirability: 3 2 1 0   Availability: 3 2 1 0

Assessment 2. Weight and height

Measure:
- Standard admission weight
- Height

STANDARD: Record at least 1 time within the first 2 days

Desirability: 3 2 1 0   Availability: 3 2 1 0

Assessment 3. Medications

Ask patient what medications he/she has been taking at home.

STANDARD: Record in medical record at least 1 time during shift patient is admitted.

Desirability: 3 2 1 0   Availability: 3 2 1 0

TABLE 2

I.   Initial Assessment (Day 1 or Day 2) Generating Nursing Data Base

PROCESS:	RATING SCALES		
	Rate the Desirability of Evaluating Each Process as a Measure of Quality 2 – Essential 1 – Preferable 0 – Unlikely to be useful Desirability of evaluating process. (Circle one)	Rate the Likelihood that the Process is Performed by Good Nurses 2 – Very likely 1 – Likely 0 – Unlikely Likelihood that process is performed. (Circle one)	Rate the Likelihood that it is Documented in the Medical Record, if the Process is Performed by Good Nurses 2 – Very likely 1 – Likely 0 – Unlikely Likelihood that process is documented. (Circle one)
Assessment 11. Skin integrity and perfusion			
Observe or examine for:			
Skin integrity, e.g. turgor, erythema, decubitis	2 1 0	2 1 0	2 1 0
Signs of perfusion, e.g., cyanosis, pallor, or temperature	2 1 0	2 1 0	2 1 0
Assessment 12. Patient's knowledge of his or her condition			
Unless unable to communicate, ask patient for his or her::			
Understanding of reason for hospitalization and/or chief complaint	2 1 0	2 1 0	2 1 0
Assessment 13. Orientation to hospital environment			
Inform patient and family about environment:			
• How to call a nurse, call light	2 1 0	2 1 0	2 1 0
• Use of side rails			
Assessment 14. Family situation, living arrangements			
Ask about:			
Preadmission residence (home, nursing home)	2 1 0	2 1 0	2 1 0
Family members and significant others	2 1 0	2 1 0	2 1 0

TABLE 3

NURSE REVIEWER BACKGROUND:

HOSPITAL EMPLOYMENT[1]

	REVIEWERS	
HOSPITAL TYPE	**#**	**%**
Teaching Hospital	10	100
Staff Model HMO[2] Hospital	1	10
City or County Hospital	4	40
Veterans Health Administration Hospital	3	30
Other Non-Profit Hospital	6	60
For-Profit Hospital	3	30
Rural Hospital	2	20

[1] Source: Responses to the Nurse Background Form question, "In what types of hospitals have you been employed for at least six months or more?" Respondents were told to check all that applied.

[2] Health Maintenance Organization

TABLE 4

NURSE REVIEWER BACKGROUND:

TYPES OF CARE[1]

	REVIEWERS WITH EACH TYPE OF EXPERIENCE							
	Direct Patient Care		Supervising Staff Care of Patients		Consulting or Educating Staff		Other Experience	
TYPE OF CARE	#	%	#	%	#	%	#	%
Geriatrics	6	60	5	50	6	60	1	10
Rehab[2]	3	30	2	20	2	20	1	10
CHF[3]	8	80	6	60	7	70	0	0
CVA[4]	6	60	5	50	6	60	1	10
ICU[5]	6	60	3	30	5	50	1	10
CCU[6]	5	50	3	30	5	50	1	10
Other	4	40	4	40	5	50	1	10

[1] Source: Responses to the Nurse Background Form question, "In the past ten years, have you had at least six months experience in the following?" Respondents were told to check every experiences that applied.

[2] Rehabilitation

[3] Congestive Heart Failure

[4] Cerebrovascular Accident

[5] Intensive Care Unit

[6] Clinical Care Unit

TABLE 5

NURSE REVIEWER BACKGROUND:
QUALITY OF CARE REVIEWS[1]

	REVIEWERS WITH EACH TYPE OF EXPERIENCE							
	At Your Hospital		For a Review Organization Like a PRO[2]		For Research		For a Hospital Chain or Region	
TYPE OF EXPERIENCE	#	%	#	%	#	%	#	%
Performed formal record reviews (i.e., chart audits) for quality assurance	6	60	2	20	4	40	0	0
Performed formal record reviews (i.e., chart audits), for utilization review	4	40	2	20	3	30	0	0
Supervised chart reviews by other abstractors	2	20	2	20	3	30	0	0
Developed quality review criteria or methods	6	60	2	20	2	20	0	0
Developed critical paths	6	60	0	0	0	0	1	10
Other	3	30	1	10	1	10	1	10

[1] Source: Responses to the Nurse Background Form question, "In the past ten years, have you had at least six months experience working with quality assurance, quality improvement, quality review, utilization review, or other kind of quality of care assessment?" Respondents were told to check all that applied.

[2] Professional Review Organization

TABLE 6

ASPECTS OF NURSING CARE REVIEWED

BY DAYS OF THE HOSPITALIZATION

Aspects of Nursing Care Reviewed:	Inpatient Hospitalization				
	Days 1 & 2	Interim Days		Day of Discharge +1 Day Prior	All Days For Other Questions
		Days 3-10 or To 1 Day Prior To Discharge, Whichever Comes First	Days 1-5 or Days 2-6		
Assessment Initial Reassessment Pre-Discharge Assessment	Q1, col II	Q1, col III	Q2	Q1, col IV	Q7
Problem Identification	Q3 Q5A				
Problem Management Goal Statement Interventions Evaluation			Q5B Q5C Q6 Q5D		
Overall Quality Measures					Q14 Q15 Q16 Q17
Other Acuity/Severity Expected Outcome Adverse Events Charting	Q4 Q10 Q11 Q12 Q13A Q13B	Q10 Q11 Q12		Q10 Q11 Q12 Q13A	Q8 Q9 Q7 Q18 Q19

APPENDIX A

NURSING BACKGROUND FORM

NURSING BACKGROUND FORM

1. In what types of hospitals have you been employed *for at least six months or more?*
   (Please check all that apply.)

   ☐ 1　Teaching hospital　　　　　　　　　　☐ 5　Other non-profit hospital

   ☐ 2　Staff model HMO, e.g., Kaiser, Cigna　☐ 6　For-profit hospital

   ☐ 3　City or county hospital　　　　　　　☐ 7　Rural hospital

   ☐ 4　Veterans Health Administration Hospital　☐ 8　Other -- > Please specify

   _____

   _____

2. *In the past ten years,* have you had *at least six months experience* in the following?
   (Please check every experience that applies.)

Type of Care	Type of Experience			
	Direct Patient Care	Supervising Staff Care of Patients	Consulting or Educating Staff	Other Experience
Geriatrics	☐ 1	☐ 2	☐ 3	☐ 4
Rehab	☐ 5	☐ 6	☐ 7	☐ 8
CHF	☐ 9	☐ 10	☐ 11	☐ 12
CVA	☐ 13	☐ 14	☐ 15	☐ 16
ICU	☐ 17	☐ 18	☐ 19	☐ 20
CCU	☐ 21	☐ 22	☐ 23	☐ 24
Other	☐ 25	☐ 26	☐ 27	☐ 28

3. *In the past ten years,* have you had *at least six months experience* working with quality assurance, quality improvement, quality review, utilization review, or other kind of quality of care assessment? *(Please check all that apply.)*

Type of Experience	Type of Experience			
	At Your Hospital	For a Review Organization Like a PRO	For Research	For a Hospital Chain or Region
Performed formal record reviews, i.e., chart audits, for quality assurance	☐ 1	☐ 2	☐ 3	☐ 4
Performed formal record reviews, i.e., chart audits, for utilization review	☐ 5	☐ 6	☐ 7	☐ 8
Supervised chart reviews by other abstractors	☐ 9	☐ 10	☐ 11	☐ 12
Developed quality review criteria or methods	☐ 13	☐ 14	☐ 15	☐ 16
Developed critical paths	☐ 17	☐ 18	☐ 19	☐ 20
Other	☐ 21	☐ 22	☐ 23	☐ 24

NURSING BACKGROUND FORM (continued)

4. Other Information:

YOUR NAME:

_____

MAILING ADDRESS:

_____

_____

PHONE(S):

(_____)_____

(_____)_____

FAX:

_____

DATE:

_____

CURRENT EMPLOYER:

_____

TITLE(S):

_____

_____

DEGREE(S):

_____

_____

DATE OF FIRST RN LICENSURE:

_____

ETHNICITY (OPTIONAL):

_____

APPENDIX B

CONGESTIVE HEART FAILURE

IMPLICIT REVIEW FORM

NINR Grant
No. RO1 NRO3681-01

RAND/UCLA

NURSING QUALITY OF CARE STUDY

IMPLICIT REVIEW

CONGESTIVE HEART FAILURE

Lisa V. Rubenstein, M.D.
Betty L. Chang, D.N.Sc., R.N.
Katherine L. Kahn, M.D.
Jan L. Lee, Ph.D, R.N.
Marjorie L. Pearson, Ph.D.

RAND
1700 Main Street
Santa Monica, CA 90407

For
The National Institute
of Nursing Research

Revised December 7, 1994

NQOC

CARD 01 7-8/

-31-

1-6/

9-14/

15-16/

17-22/

23-25/

CARD 01

NURSING QUALITY OF CARE STUDY
IMPLICIT REVIEW FORM

CONGESTIVE HEART FAILURE

ADMINISTRATIVE DATA

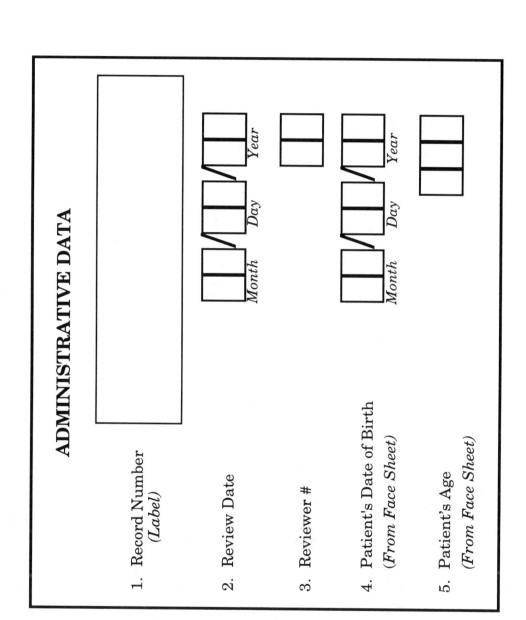

1. Record Number
   (Label)

2. Review Date

   Month / Day / Year

3. Reviewer #

4. Patient's Date of Birth
   (From Face Sheet)

   Month / Day / Year

5. Patient's Age
   (From Face Sheet)

NURSING QUALITY OF CARE STUDY (CHF)

1. HEALTH STATUS AND NEEDS ASSESSMENT: DATA GATHERING

Please rate the quality of nurses' assessment for each of the items listed in Column I. In rating each assessment, consider both the frequency and type of data collection needed in relation to the patient's condition. To understand the patient's condition, use the whole medical record. To judge the quality of nurse assessment, use only data recorded by nurses. For more information on the rating scale, see the section on Question 1 in your Instruction Manual.

Column I Assessment Item	Column II Initial Assessment					Column III Reassessment					Column IV Pre-discharge Assessment				
For each item below, circle one number in each column across (Columns II, III & IV).	*Base your rating on day 1 and day 2 of this hospitalization (total of 2 days).*					*Base your rating on day 3 to day 10 (total of 8 days), or to one day prior to discharge, whichever comes first.* ☐ *Check here if patient died prior to day 4. If so, leave this column blank.*					*Base your rating on day of discharge plus one day prior to discharge for this hospitalization (total of 2 days).* ☐ *Check here if patient died in hospital. If so, leave this column blank.*				
	Excel-lent	Good	Ade-quate	Poor	Very Poor	Excel-lent	Good	Ade-quate	Poor	Very Poor	Excel-lent	Good	Ade-quate	Poor	Very Poor
	(1)	(2)	(3)	(4)	(5)	(1)	(2)	(3)	(4)	(5)	(1)	(2)	(3)	(4)	(5)
A. General Health Status Assessment for Communicative and Non-communicative Patients	(Circle One Number)					(Circle One Number)					(Circle One Number)				
a) Vital signs	1	2	3	4	5	1	2	3	4	5	1	2	3	4	5
b) Weight	1	2	3	4	5	1	2	3	4	5	1	2	3	4	5
c) Pre-hospital medications	1	2	3	4	5										
d) Allergies	1	2	3	4	5										

26-27/ 28-30/ 31-33/ 34/ 35/

NURSING QUALITY OF CARE STUDY (CHF)

1. (Continued) HEALTH STATUS AND NEEDS ASSESSMENT: DATA GATHERING
(See page 2 for wording of question)

Column I Assessment Item	Column II Initial Assessment					Column III Reassessment					Column IV Pre-discharge Assessment					
For each item below, circle one number in each column across (Columns II, III & IV).	*Base your rating on day 1 and day 2 of this hospitalization (total of 2 days).*					*Base your rating on day 3 to day 10 (total of 8 days), or to one day prior to discharge, whichever comes first.*					*Base your rating on day of discharge plus one day prior to discharge for this hospitalization (total of 2 days).*					
						Reminder: *This column is to be left blank if patient died prior to day 4.*					**Reminder:** *This column is to be left blank if patient died in hospital.*					
	Excel-lent	Good	Ade-quate	Poor	Very Poor	Excel-lent	Good	Ade-quate	Poor	Very Poor	Excel-lent	Good	Ade-quate	Poor	Very Poor	
	(1)	(2)	(3)	(4)	(5)	(1)	(2)	(3)	(4)	(5)	(1)	(2)	(3)	(4)	(5)	
A. (Continued) **General Health Status Assessment for Communicative and Non-communicative Patients**	(Circle One Number)					(Circle One Number)					(Circle One Number)					
e) Communication (*e.g. speech*), and sensory abilities (*e.g. eyesight, hearing, need for aids*)	1	2	3	4	5	1	2	3	4	5	1	2	3	4	5	36-38/
f) Physical functional status (*e.g., walking, eating, bathing, toileting*) and activity tolerance (*e.g., getting out of bed, walking*)	1	2	3	4	5	1	2	3	4	5	1	2	3	4	5	39-41/
g) Rest (*e.g., sleep, agitation*)	1	2	3	4	5	1	2	3	4	5	1	2	3	4	5	42-44/

NURSING QUALITY OF CARE STUDY (CHF)

1. (Continued) HEALTH STATUS AND NEEDS ASSESSMENT: DATA GATHERING
(See page 2 for wording of question)

Column I Assessment Item	Column II Initial Assessment					Column III Reassessment					Column IV Pre-discharge Assessment				
For each item below, circle one number in each column across (Columns II, III & IV).	*Base your rating on day 1 and day 2 of this hospitalization (total of 2 days).*					*Base your rating on day 3 to day 10 (total of 8 days), or to one day prior to discharge, whichever comes first.* **Reminder:** *This column is to be left blank if patient died prior to day 4.*					*Base your rating on day of discharge plus one day prior to discharge for this hospitalization (total of 2 days).* **Reminder:** *This column is to be left blank if patient died in hospital.*				
	Excel-lent (1)	Good (2)	Ade-quate (3)	Poor (4)	Very Poor (5)	Excel-lent (1)	Good (2)	Ade-quate (3)	Poor (4)	Very Poor (5)	Excel-lent (1)	Good (2)	Ade-quate (3)	Poor (4)	Very Poor (5)
	(Circle One Number)					(Circle One Number)					(Circle One Number)				
A. (Continued) **General Health Status Assessment for Communicative and Non-communicative Patients**															
h) Mental status (*e.g., alertness, orientation*)	1	2	3	4	5	1	2	3	4	5	1	2	3	4	5
i) Pain	1	2	3	4	5	1	2	3	4	5	1	2	3	4	5
j) Nutritional intake and diet (*e.g., type of diet, amount of food, food preferences*)	1	2	3	4	5	1	2	3	4	5	1	2	3	4	5
k) Bowel and bladder function (*e.g., frequency, quantity, continence/incontinence*)	1	2	3	4	5	1	2	3	4	5	1	2	3	4	5

45–47/
48–50/
51–53/
54–56/

NURSING QUALITY OF CARE STUDY (CHF)

1. (Continued)   HEALTH STATUS AND NEEDS ASSESSMENT: DATA GATHERING
(See page 2 for wording of question)

Column I Assessment Item	Column II Initial Assessment					Column III Reassessment					Column IV Pre-discharge Assessment					
For each item below, circle one number in each column across (Columns II, III & IV).	*Base your rating on day 1 and day 2 of this hospitalization (total of 2 days).*					*Base your rating on day 3 to day 10 (total of 8 days), or to one day prior to discharge, whichever comes first.* **Reminder:** *This column is to be left blank if patient died prior to day 4.*					*Base your rating on day of discharge plus one day prior to discharge for this hospitalization (total of 2 days).* **Reminder:** *This column is to be left blank if patient died in hospital.*					
	Excel-lent	Good	Ade-quate	Poor	Very Poor	Excel-lent	Good	Ade-quate	Poor	Very Poor	Excel-lent	Good	Ade-quate	Poor	Very Poor	
	(1)	(2)	(3)	(4)	(5)	(1)	(2)	(3)	(4)	(5)	(1)	(2)	(3)	(4)	(5)	
A. (Continued) **General Health Status Assessment for Communicative and Non-communicative Patients**	(Circle One Number)					(Circle One Number)					(Circle One Number)					
l) Skin condition (*e.g., integrity, moisture, turgor, color*)	1	2	3	4	5	1	2	3	4	5	1	2	3	4	5	57–59/
m) Out of hospital living arrangements	1	2	3	4	5						1	2	3	4	5	60–61/
n) Family/significant other involvement with patient (*e.g., who is notified in emergencies; who makes decisions regarding patient; social contacts*)	1	2	3	4	5	1	2	3	4	5	1	2	3	4	5	62–64/

CARD 01

NURSING QUALITY OF CARE STUDY (CHF)

1. (Continued) HEALTH STATUS AND NEEDS ASSESSMENT: DATA GATHERING
(See page 2 for wording of question)

Column I Assessment Item For each item below, circle one number in each column across (Columns II, III & IV). ☐ Check here if patient does not communicate with speech. If so, go to C (next page).	Column II Initial Assessment Base your rating on day 1 and day 2 of this hospitalization (total of 2 days).					Column III Reassessment Base your rating on day 3 to day 10 (total of 8 days), or to one day prior to discharge, whichever comes first. Reminder: This column is to be left blank if patient died prior to day 4					Column IV Pre-discharge Assessment Base your rating on day of discharge plus one day prior to discharge for this hospitalization (total of 2 days). Reminder: This column is to be left blank if patient died in hospital.				
	Excel- lent (1)	Good (2)	Ade- quate (3)	Poor (4)	Very Poor (5)	Excel- lent (1)	Good (2)	Ade- quate (3)	Poor (4)	Very Poor (5)	Excel- lent (1)	Good (2)	Ade- quate (3)	Poor (4)	Very Poor (5)
B. General Health Status Assessment for Communicative Patients Only	(Circle One Number)					(Circle One Number)					(Circle One Number)				
a) Psychological state (e.g., mood)	1	2	3	4	5	1	2	3	4	5	1	2	3	4	5
b) Patient's knowledge of his/her condition and medications (e.g., patient identifies own health problems, patient counseled prior to discharge)	1	2	3	4	5	1	2	3	4	5	1	2	3	4	5
c) Orientation to physical hospital environment (e.g., bells, rails, telephone, visitors)	1	2	3	4	5										

9-11/

12-14/

15/

CARD 02

NURSING QUALITY OF CARE STUDY (CHF)

1. (Continued) HEALTH STATUS AND NEEDS ASSESSMENT: DATA GATHERING

(See page 2 for wording of question)

Column I Assessment Item	Column II Initial Assessment					Column III Reassessment					Column IV Pre-discharge Assessment					
For each item below, circle one number in each column across (Columns II, III & IV).	Base your rating on day 1 and day 2 of this hospitalization (total of 2 days).					Base your rating on day 3 to day 10 (total of 8 days), or to one day prior to discharge, whichever comes first. *Reminder: This column is to be left blank if patient died prior to day 4.*					Base your rating on day of discharge plus one day prior to discharge for this hospitalization (total of 2 days). *Reminder: This column is to be left blank if patient died in hospital.*					
	Excel- lent (1)	Good (2)	Ade- quate (3)	Poor (4)	Very Poor (5)	Excel- lent (1)	Good (2)	Ade- quate (3)	Poor (4)	Very Poor (5)	Excel- lent (1)	Good (2)	Ade- quate (3)	Poor (4)	Very Poor (5)	
C. **Diagnostic-Specific Health Status Assessment for Communicative and Non-communicative Patients**	(Circle One Number)					(Circle One Number)					(Circle One Number)					
a) Cardiovascular (e.g., chest pain, cardiac exam, pedal edema)	1	2	3	4	5	1	2	3	4	5	1	2	3	4	5	16-18/
b) Respiratory (e.g., breath sounds, shortness of breath)	1	2	3	4	5	1	2	3	4	5	1	2	3	4	5	19-21/

NURSING QUALITY OF CARE STUDY (CHF)

2. PHYSICIAN ORDERS

Were physician orders which were written on day 1 and day 2 implemented by the nurses exactly as ordered (or more frequently or thoroughly) for:

(Circle One Number in Each Line)

	Yes	No/No Data	
a) Vital Signs	1	9	22/
b) Weight	1	9	23/

3. EXPLICIT IDENTIFICATION OF PROBLEMS

How often did the nurses explicitly identify problems that you regard as nursing issues for the care of this patient? (To answer this question, think about problems you identified during your review for Question 1 and assess whether nurses actually labeled these problems or listed them in some statement of problems).

(Circle One Number)

All or Many Problems Stated	About Half of Problems Stated	Some Problems Stated	No Problems Stated	
1	2	3	4	24/

4. NEED FOR NURSING INTERVENTION

Please rate the amount (i.e., quantity and intensity) of nursing intervention needed to provide optimal care for this patient. (To do this, think again about problems you identified during your review of days 1 and 2 for Question 1, and what you would do to manage them). Focus on what the patient needed, not on what the patient got.

(Circle One Number)

Above Average Amount of Nursing Interventions	About Average Amount of Nursing Interventions	Below Average Amount of Nursing Interventions	
1	2	3	25/

5. MANAGEMENT OF PROBLEMS

Please rate the quality of nurses' management for each tracer problem that applies to this patient.

5A.
Did the patient have this problem?

For items in 5A.1, review Actual Tracer Problem from day 1 and day 2 of the medical record.

IF NO *to any problem, go to next problem.*

IF YES *to any problem, answer Questions 5B-5D across, before going to next problem.*

5B.
Were any nursing goals, expected outcomes, or planned actions explicitly stated for this problem?

Base your answer on nursing notes from the day the problem occurred through the subsequent 4 days (total of 5 days).

5C.
Were appropriate nursing interventions for this problem carried out?

Base your answer on nursing notes from the day the problem occurred through the subsequent 4 days (total of 5 days).

5D.
Is the nurses' record ever explicit about whether the patient's problem improved, worsened or stayed the same?

Base your answer on nursing notes from the day the problem occurred through the subsequent 4 days (total of 5 days).

PROBLEM 5A.1 Actual Tracer Problem (Identified from Day 1 & Day 2 Records)	5A. No/ No Data (9)	5A. Yes (1)	5B. Yes (1)	5B. No (9)	5C. Yes, All (1)	5C. Yes, Most (2)	5C. Yes, Some (3)	5C. No, None (4)	5D. Yes (1)	5D. No (9)	
	(Circle One Number)		(Circle One Number)		(Circle One Number)				(Circle One Number)		
a) Fever	9	1→	1	9	1	2	3	4	1	9	26-29/
b) Diabetes	9	1→	1	9	1	2	3	4	1	9	30-33/
c) Anxiety or Depression	9	1→	1	9	1	2	3	4	1	9	34-37/
d) Self-care deficit with feeding	9	1→	1	9	1	2	3	4	1	9	38-41/
e) Impaired physical mobility including activity intolerance (e.g., shortness of breath with walking)	9	1→	1	9	1	2	3	4	1	9	42-45/

NURSING QUALITY OF CARE STUDY (CHF)

5. (Continued) MANAGEMENT OF PROBLEMS

PROBLEM 5A.1 (continued) Actual Tracer Problem (Identified from Day 1 & Day 2 Records)	5A. Did the patient have this problem? For items in 5A.1, review Actual Tracer Problems from day 1 and day 2 of the medical record. IF NO to any problem, go to next problem. IF YES to any problem, answer Questions 5B–5D across, before going to next problem.		5B. Were any nursing goals, expected outcomes, or planned actions explicitly stated for this problem? Base your answer on nursing notes from the day the problem occurred through the subsequent 4 days (total of 5 days).		5C. Were appropriate nursing interventions for this problem carried out? Base your answer on nursing notes from the day the problem occurred through the subsequent 4 days (total of 5 days).				5D. Is the nurse's record ever explicit about whether the patient's problem improved, worsened or stayed the same? Base your answer on nursing notes from the day the problem occurred through the subsequent 4 days (total of 5 days).		
	No/ No Data (9)	Yes (1)	Yes (1)	No (9)	Yes, All (1)	Yes, Most (2)	Yes, Some (3)	No, None (4)	Yes (1)	No (9)	
	(Circle One Number)		(Circle One Number)		(Circle One Number)				(Circle One Number)		
f) Shock or blood pressure ≤ 90	9	1→	1	9	1	2	3	4	1	9	46–49/
g) Chest Pain	9	1→	1	9	1	2	3	4	1	9	50–53/
h) Non-cardiac pain	9	1→	1	9	1	2	3	4	1	9	54–57/
i) Knowledge deficit regarding his/her condition and medication (if patient does not communicate with speech, circle '9'; otherwise circle '1' since all patients require some education about their condition and medication)	9	1→	1	9	1	2	3	4	1	9	58–61/

NURSING QUALITY OF CARE STUDY (CHF)

5. (Continued) MANAGEMENT OF PROBLEMS

5A.
Did the patient have this problem?

For items in 5A.2, review Actual or Potential Tracer Problems from day 1 and day 2 of the medical record.

IF NO to any problem, go to next problem.

IF YES to any problem, answer Questions 5B-5D across, before going to next problem.

5B.
Were any nursing goals, expected outcomes or planned actions explicitly stated for this problem?

Base your answer on nursing notes from the day the problem occurred through the subsequent 4 days (total of 5 days).

5C.
Were appropriate nursing interventions for this problem carried out?

Base your answer on nursing notes from the day the problem occurred through the subsequent 4 days (total of 5 days).

5D.
Is the nurse's record ever explicit about whether the patient's problem improved, worsened or stayed the same?

Base your answer on nursing notes from the day the problem occurred through the subsequent 4 days (total of 5 days).

PROBLEM 5A.2 — Actual or Potential Tracer Problem (Identified from Day 1 & Day 2 Records)	5A — No/No Data (9)	5A — Yes (1)	5B — Yes (1)	5B — No (9)	5C — Yes, All (1)	5C — Yes, Most (2)	5C — Yes, Some (3)	5C — No, None (4)	5D — Yes (1)	5D — No (9)
	(Circle One Number)		(Circle One Number)		(Circle One Number)				(Circle One Number)	
a) Pulmonary edema/pulmonary congestion (e.g., high respiratory rate, rapid pulse, shortness of breath)	9	1→	1	9	1	2	3	4	1	9
b) Actual or high risk for impaired skin integrity (e.g., incontinent, limited bed or chair mobility, poorly nourished, comatose, edematous, or actual or suspected decubitus)	9	1→	1	9	1	2	3	4	1	9

NURSING QUALITY OF CARE STUDY (CHF)

5. (Continued) MANAGEMENT OF PROBLEMS

5A.
Did the patient have this problem?

For items in 5A.2, review Actual or Potential Tracer Problems from day 1 and day 2 of the medical record.

IF NO to any problem, go to next problem.

IF YES to any problem, answer Questions 5B-5D across, before going to next problem.

5B.
Were any nursing goals, expected outcomes, or planned actions explicitly stated for this problem?

Base your answer on nursing notes from the day the problem occurred through the subsequent 4 days (total of 5 days).

5C.
Were appropriate nursing interventions for this problem carried out?

Base your answer on nursing notes from the day the problem occurred through the subsequent 4 days (total of 5 days).

5D.
Is the nurse's record ever explicit about whether the patient's problem improved, worsened or stayed the same?

Base your answer on nursing notes from the day the problem occurred through the subsequent 4 days (total of 5 days).

PROBLEM 5A.2 (continued) Actual or Potential Tracer Problem (Identified from Day 1 & Day 2 Records)	5A. No/ No Data (9)	5A. Yes (1)	5B. Yes (1)	5B. No (9)	5C. Yes, All (1)	5C. Yes, Most (2)	5C. Yes, Some (3)	5C. No, None (4)	5D. Yes (1)	5D. No (9)
	(Circle One Number)		(Circle One Number)		(Circle One Number)				(Circle One Number)	
c) Dysrhythmias (e.g., irregular pulse)	9	1→	1	9	1	2	3	4	1	9
d) High risk for injury secondary to confusion	9	1→	1	9	1	2	3	4	1	9
e) Other (Specify): _____	9	1→	1	9	1	2	3	4	1	9

17-20/

21-24/

25-28/

CARD 03

NURSING QUALITY OF CARE STUDY (CHF)

5. (Continued) MANAGEMENT OF PROBLEMS

PROBLEM 5A.3	**5A.** Does the patient have this problem? *For items in 5A.3, review Vital Signs Flowsheets from day 3 and after.* **IF NO** *go to Question 6.* **IF YES** *answer Questions 5B-5D across.*		**5B.** Were any nursing goals, expected outcomes, or planned actions explicitly stated for this problem? *Base your answer on nursing notes from the day the problem occurred through the subsequent 4 days (total of 5 days).*		**5C.** Were appropriate nursing interventions for this problem carried out? *Base your answer on nursing notes from the day the problem occurred through the subsequent 4 days (total of 5 days).*				**5D.** Is the nurse's record explicit about whether the patient's problem improved, worsened or stayed the same? *Base your answer on nursing notes from the day the problem occurred through the subsequent 4 days (total of 5 days).*	
Change in Status *(Identified from Vital Signs Flowsheets from Day 3 or After)*	No/ No Data (9)	Yes (1) →	Yes (1)	No (9)	Yes, All (1)	Yes, Most (2)	Yes, Some (3)	No, None (4)	Yes (1)	No (9)
	(Circle One Number)		(Circle One Number)		(Circle One Number)				(Circle One Number)	
a) Change in vital signs *(i.e., blood pressure, respiration, temperature, pulse)*	9	1 →	1	9	1	2	3	4	1	9

NURSING QUALITY OF CARE STUDY (CHF)

6. APPROPRIATENESS OF INTERVENTIONS

Whether or not all the problems detected as you reviewed the medical record were explicitly recorded by nurses, rate the degree to which the nurses <u>carried out</u> the appropriate interventions for all these problems, (including changing the frequency of monitoring). Use the data sources for Questions 1 and 4.

(Circle One Number)

All or Most <u>Carried Out</u>	About Half <u>Carried Out</u>	Some <u>Carried Out</u>	Few or None <u>Carried Out</u>
1	2	3	4

33/

7. QUALITY OF MEDICATION ADMINISTRATION DOCUMENTATION

What is the quality of nurses' documentation related to medication administration and actual or potential medication side effects? Use medication records and nurses' notes.

(Circle One Number)

<u>Excellent</u>	<u>Good</u>	<u>Fair</u>	<u>Poor</u>
1	2	3	4

34/

NURSING QUALITY OF CARE STUDY (CHF)

8. ADVERSE NURSING EVENTS

Did any of the following adverse nursing events occur during this hospitalization? Use special reports and data sources you have already reviewed for Questions 1 and 4, i.e., days 1 through 10, if applicable, and the day of and day prior to discharge.

(Circle One Number on Each Line)

	Yes	No/No Data	
a) Medication Error.........................	1	9	35/
b) Fall.........................	1	9	36/
c) Underdosing of a PRN Medication.........	1	9	37/
d) Overdosing of a PRN Medication.........	1	9	38/
e) Patient Discharged Unstable *(Circle '9' if patient died)*.........	1	9	39/
f) Other *(Specify)* _____	1	9	40/

8A. **REVIEWER INSTRUCTIONS**

- *If you answered Yes to any item in Question 8 above, underline Question 9.*
- *If you answered No/No Data to every item (a-f) in Question 8, above, go to Question 10.*

NURSING QUALITY OF CARE STUDY (CHF)

9. ADVERSE EVENT MANAGEMENT

(Answer if you circled YES to any adverse event in Question 8)

Rate how well the nurse managed the problem. (IF more than one problem, rate the first one circled YES on the list).

(Circle One Number)

Extremely Well	Well	Adequately	Poorly	Very Poorly
1	2	3	4	5

41/

10. NEED FOR NURSING TIME

How much nursing time would it take to provide optimal care to the patient described in this medical record, compared to most congestive heart failure patients?

(Circle One Number)

More than Average Time	Average Time	Less than Average Time
1	2	3

42/

11. NEED FOR NURSING EXPERTISE

How much nursing expertise would it take to provide optimal care to the patient described in this medical record, compared to most congestive heart failure patients?

(Circle One Number)

More than Average Expertise	Average Expertise	Less than Average Expertise
1	2	3

43/

CARD 03

12. NEED FOR NURSING SPECIAL TRAINING

How much could this patient benefit from care by a nurse with special training in geriatrics or cardiology, compared to care by nurses without this special training?

(Circle One Number)

Greatly Benefit	Somewhat Benefit	Little or No Benefit
1	2	3

44/

13. PATIENT DISCHARGE

(IF patient was discharged alive, ANSWER 13A. IF patient was discharged dead, ANSWER 13B).

13A. *PATIENT WAS DISCHARGED ALIVE: How would you characterize the patient's condition at discharge, given this patient's status at admission (hospital days 1 and 2)?*

(Circle One Number)

Much Better Than Expected	Better Than Expected	As Expected	Worse Than Expected	Much Worse Than Expected
1	2	3	4	5

45/

13B. *PATIENT WAS DISCHARGED DEAD: How would you characterize the death, given this patient's status at admission (hospital days 1 and 2)?*

(Circle One Number)

Definitely Expected	Somewhat Expected	Somewhat Unexpected	Definitely Unexpected
1	2	3	4

46/

NURSING QUALITY OF CARE STUDY (CHF)

14. QUALITY OF PATIENT SERVICES

How would you characterize the quality of the following services delivered to this patient?

(Circle One Number in Each Line)

	Excellent	Good	Fair	Poor	
a) Nursing care	1	2	3	4	47/
b) Physician care	1	2	3	4	48/

15. OVERALL QUALITY OF CARE

Considering everything you know about this patient, please rate overall quality of care.

(Circle One Number)

Extreme, Above Standard	Above Standard	Adequate	Below Standard	Extreme, Below Standard	
1	2	3	4	5	49/

16. RATING OF NURSES

Would you want your mother cared for by these nurses in this hospital?

(Circle One Number)

Definitely Yes	Probably Yes	Probably No	Definitely No	
1	2	3	4	50/

CARD 03

NURSING QUALITY OF CARE STUDY (CHF)

17. RATING OF PHYSICIANS

Would you want your mother cared for by these physicians in this hospital?

(Circle One Number)

Definitely Yes	Probably Yes	Probably No	Definitely No
1	2	3	4

9/

18. CHARTING METHODS

18A. *Which of the following charting methods were used in this medical record?*

(Circle All that Apply)

Nurses notes (without problem focus)	1
Problem Oriented Method of Recording (POMR)	2
Preprinted nursing care plans, (e.g., standard care plans)	3
On-line computerized forms excluding nursing care plans, (e.g., computerized medication forms)	4
On-line computerized nursing care plans................................	5
Charting by exception................................	6
Other (Specify): _____	7

10/

11/

12/

13/

14/

15/

16/

18B. *Of the methods circled above, which **one** method was used the **most** to record information about the type and course of the patient's nursing problems or diagnoses and interventions? (In the box below, please enter the number from Question 18A that corresponds to your answer).*

17/

NURSING QUALITY OF CARE STUDY (CHF)

19. ADDITIONAL FORMS

In addition to medication, IV, TPR, ICU, and intake & output flowsheet records, which of the following were present in this record?

(Circle all that apply)

Activity, functional status, or neurological record (sheet) 1   18/

Disease or condition oriented sheet (e.g., diabetes or pressure ulcer record) 2   19/

Other specialized sheet (e.g., teaching record) 3   20/

Form resembling patient Kardex or care plan sheet (e.g., form with columns for problem list, interventions, and dates) 4   21/

20. COMMENTS

_____

_____   22-24/

_____

Please carefully review each page of this form to insure that all questions are answered.

APPENDIX C

CONGESTIVE HEART FAILURE
IMPLICIT REVIEW INSTRUCTIONS

NURSING QUALITY OF CARE STUDY
STRUCTURED IMPLICIT REVIEW
CONGESTIVE HEART FAILURE

INSTRUCTIONS

General Approach to Implicit Review:

1.) *Thinking about outcomes:*

When you judge the quality of nursing care, think about the probability that the care given maximized (or worsened) the chance that the patient would experience a good outcome, whatever the actual outcome was. For example, out of 100 patients in the same clinical state as the patient under review, how many would have suffered an adverse outcome if treated this way, compared to the number who would have done so if treated optimally? If the likelihood of an adverse outcome is significantly increased by deficiencies in the care delivered, we judge the care to be poor. If the likelihood of an adverse outcome is minimized, we judge care to be excellent.

2.) *Thinking about health care providers and judgments about quality:*

In judging the quality of the process of nursing care, we are interested in whether the patient's needs were met. We do not try to assign blame or find reasons for omissions, nor to assess how difficult or easy it was to meet the patient's needs. If the patient received what was needed, the care should be judged as excellent, even if he or she did not need much. Likewise, if the patient did not receive what was needed, the care should be judged as poor, whether or not the case was difficult. Your ratings should not be affected if more care is given than needed unless the extra care is harmful. Do not judge care differently depending upon whether you think the patient came from a rural, urban, county or other type of hospital. Think about the level of care achievable by good but not extraordinary hospitals and judge care accordingly.

3.) *Judging 1981-1986 Medical Records*:

If standards have changed over the past decade for a particular aspect of care, use your recollection of early to mid-1980's standards for assessing what a patient needed. If standards remained the same but practice changed due to technological advances, use 1980's practices to judge whether the patient received what he or she needed. On the other hand, if standards remained the same while nursing practice changed, but not due to technological advances, base your judgments on current practice. Skin integrity care presents an example of the latter situation in that standards were the same in the 1980's as now, although a general perception is that adherence to these standards has improved significantly over time. We can therefore judge 1980's care by current standards.

4.) *Making Inferences from the Record*:

Reviewers often want to give the "benefit of the doubt" in judging care by inferring what might have happened to explain the way care was delivered. Here too keep in mind that we are interested in whether the patient's needs were met, not in establishing blame or reasons for problems. Do not infer actions or events, but, rather, judge solely on the basis of the record. Ignore the fact that some information, such as information in the Cardex, may not be present in the record. The research team will make it clear in reporting the results of this project that the Cardex was not available.

5.) *Thinking about Patients Who Have "Do Not Resuscitate" Orders*:

We ask that you not take account of these orders in judging the quality of nursing care for the records you will review by lowering your expectations about the assessments and interventions needed. Make your judgments solely on the basis of what the person needs. During this time period, whether or not a person received a "do not resuscitate order" (DNR) may have been rather arbitrary. We will identify and take account of the DNR patients in the data analysis. We also can take account of the functionally impaired and very old patients who did not receive DNR orders but may have been implicitly treated as if they did.

6. *The role of the implicit reviewer*:

      Implicit reviewers are the "gold standard" expert reviewers of medical records. Experts do not always agree on what should be done, so we expect some variation between reviewer judgments. In implicit review, however, a significant amount of variation can come from differences in the data sources used, in the interpretation of rating scales, and in the understanding of the types of quality being assessed. We attempt to reduce variation due to arbitrary methodological differences such as those due to rating scales and data sources, while continuing to allow for true differences of opinion between reviewers.

7.) *Organizing the Review and Filling Out the Front Page*:

      We suggest that you first familiarize yourself with the structured implicit review form. Then, follow these Instructions for answering specific items on the form.

      Prior to reviewing the patient record, please check that the record number on the label on the Implicit Review Form is the same as the record number on the medical record. Then write the date on which you are reviewing the case, your reviewer number, the patient's date of birth, and the patient's age on the first page of the form. If the information is missing, enter 9 in the appropriate boxes.

      Begin your review of the medical record by reviewing the physician's notes and recording any major adverse events or nursing relevant diagnoses on the worksheet provided. This may alert you to key issues in the patient's care to look for while reviewing the more lengthy nursing notes.

      Then review all of the data recorded by nurses, including narrative notes, flow sheets, medication, care plans, etc. for the days indicated in the instructions. We suggest that you answer Question 1 as you read, while recording key events on your worksheet. Then go back to the important dates to answer subsequent questions. Feel free to write notes in the medical record as you proceed and/or mark significant areas with post-its.

QUESTION 1. Health Status and Needs Assessment: Data Gathering

Please rate the quality of nurse assessment for each of the items listed in Column 1. In rating each assessment, consider both the frequency and type of data collection needed in relation to the patient's condition. To understand the patient's condition, use the whole medical record. To judge the quality of nurse assessment, use only data recorded by nurses.

Purpose

This question tries to determine the quality of the nursing assessment/data gathering, as reflected in the medical record. It asks whether the information is what you would need to know about the patient's status in order for you to adequately care for the patient. For each patient, pertinent positive and pertinent negatives that you believe are important may vary according to the patient's condition. Thus, the level of documentation necessary to assign a particular rating (e.g. excellent) should vary for each case since each patient's unique clinical picture will influence the amount and kind of information you believe is necessary.

Consider what data you think should be collected given the patient's needs, not what data are requested by the hospital's forms.

The word "assessment" is sometimes used to mean that the data collector understands and analyzes the data. In Question 1, however, we mean the collection of data and not a judgment regarding the patient's problems. Assessment data pertaining to each topic listed can be collected by interview, physical exam, or laboratory testing. Because health status assessment is so critical to patient care, we expect that nurses will comment in the record about the presence, absence, or availability of information relevant to each item listed in Column I.

This question is divided into three parts. In Part A you are asked to rate how adequate the nurses' recordings are in allowing you to rate this patient's general health status assessment as indicated by specific items [A.a through A.n]. In Part B, you are asked to rate general health status assessment by nurses on items that are relevant only to patients who can communicate by speech. If the patient can communicate, rate items B.a through B.c. In Part C, you are asked to rate nursing assessment of specific aspects of health status particularly relevant to congestive heart failure [C.a and C.b].

These ratings should be done for three periods of the patient's hospital stay: 1) on initial assessment, 2) on reassessment, and 3) pre-discharge. By initial assessment, we mean the interview and examination of the patient upon admission. Include in your judgment whether the initial assessment was timely. By reassessment, we mean the monitoring or evaluation of the patient during his/her course of hospitalization after the initial assessment and prior to predischarge assessment. Reassessment can include both the systematic search for new problems and further data gathering about previously identified problems. By predischarge assessment, we mean the patient examination and interview performed in preparation for discharge. This assessment may be done over a period of time rather than just on the day of discharge and may be recorded in a variety of places (e.g., patient teaching forms, nurses notes, consultation notes). Again, we are interested in your judgment about whether this predischarge assessment was sufficiently timely for the patient to be discharged appropriately. If the patient died in the hospital, do not rate the quality of the predischarge assessment, i.e., leave Column IV blank. Similarly, if the patient died within the first two days of admission or was discharged alive within 4 days of admission, leave Column III blank. For example, a patient who was discharged alive on the third hospital day should be rated for initial assessment (Column II) and predischarge assessment for day 3 (Column IV); reassessment (Column III) should be left blank. A patient who died on the third hospital day should be rated for initial assessment (Column II) and reassessment for day 3 (Column III); predischarge assessment (Column IV should be left blank.

Data Sources

The data sources for rating the quality of nurse assessment (Question 1) is limited to data recorded by nurses, including nurse notes, admission and discharge notes, temperature, pulse, and respiration sheets, medication sheets,. flow sheets, and specific data sheets (e.g., patient education, skin care). You should use all data in the medical record to understand what data were needed for the patient, but use only the data recorded by nurses to actually rate the nurse assessment. For ratings in Column II (initial assessment), review days 1 and 2 of hospitalization. For ratings in Column III (reassessment), review days 3 through

10 of hospitalization, or up to the day prior to discharge. For Column IV, review the day of and the day prior to discharge.

Rating Scale

Consider the quantity, timing, and importance of the information needed, given the patient's condition.

Excellent: Assign *excellent* if, as the registered nurse caring for this patient, you would not need to collect any further data.

Good: Between *excellent* and *adequate*.

Adequate: Assign *adequate* if, as the nurse responsible for this patient, you believe you would gather some additional data.

Poor: Between *adequate* and *very poor*.

Very Poor: Assign *very poor* if, as the nurse responsible for this patient, you would collect virtually all of the information or particularly critical pieces of information from the initial assessment, reassessment, or predischarge assessment to have the information you would need.

Save the *excellent* rating for assessments that were truly excellent, i.e., that obtained all of the key information needed as often as needed. A rating of *excellent* should mean that you would not want to distinguish any better assessments. These should be exemplary assessments that could be achieved in average hospitals.

Similarly, save the worst rating for those that are truly very poor. A rating of *very poor* should mean that you would not want to distinguish any worse assessment.

Consider *adequate* as middle of the road.

SPECIFIC ITEMS

QUESTION 1, Part A. General Health Status Assessment for Communicative and Non-Communicative Patients.

Most general health status assessments are applicable to all patients with CHF whether or not they are able to communicate with the nurse (Items in A and C). Some assessments, however, such as mood, are most applicable to patients who can communicate (Items in B).

Item 1A.a. Documentation of Vital Signs.

Item 1A.a asks you to rate the frequency and timing of measurement of temperature, pulse, respiration, and blood pressure. These can be documented anywhere in the chart.

Item 1A.b. Documentation of Weight.

Item 1A.b asks about frequency and timing of measurement of the patient's weight. By <u>weight</u>, we mean how heavy the patient is in pounds or kilograms according to the patient's self-report or actual weight obtained by the nurse. In general, estimated weight should be evaluated as poorer quality than actual weight. If there is a note indicating that actually weighing the patient is very difficult or impossible, you may wish to take this into account and upgrade the rating.

Item 1A.c. Documentation of Prehospital Medications.

Item 1A.c asks you to rate the completeness of nursing documentation on <u>prehospital medications</u>, i.e., data collected on medications the patient may have been taking at home, when the last dose was taken, and any medications given on admission to the hospital.

Item 1A.d. Documentation of Allergies.

Item 1A.d asks you to rate the completeness of nursing documentation of allergies. We define <u>allergies</u> to include hyper-sensitivity to food and medications upon admission. If no allergies exist, documentation may be "no allergies known."

Item 1A.e. Documentation of Communication and Sensory Abilities.

Item 1A.e asks you to rate the completeness of nursing documentation of the patient's communication and sensory abilities. Some examples are speech defects, language, and use of glasses. Judge these records in comparison to what you think the records should contain in order to take adequate care of the patient. For example, assign an excellent rating if the record has provided you all the information necessary about communication and sensory abilities, in order to make a good nursing care plan for the patient and affect the outcomes of care in this patient. Assign an adequate rating if there is some indication that the nurses were aware of these domains but the information is significantly incomplete. Do not include mental status assessment which is covered in Item 1A.h.

Item 1A.f. Documentation of Physical Functional Status and Activity Tolerance.

Item 1A.f asks you to rate the completeness and timing of nursing documentation of the patient's functional status and activity tolerance. By functional status, we mean the patient's ability to carry on usual activities of daily life, such as eating, dressing, bathing, or toileting. Activity tolerance relates to the patient's ability to withstand activities, such as getting out of bed, going to the bathroom, being up in a chair, walking. Please note that toileting does not refer to the patient's continence but, rather, to the patient's ability to use a toilet, commode, urinal, or bedpan.

Item 1A.g. Documentation of Rest.

Item 1A.g asks you to rate the completeness and timeliness of nursing documentation regarding quality, quantity, presence or absence of the patient's rest. By rest, we mean that the records should contain data for you to judge whether or not the patient rested well during the day or night, slept, or appeared agitated.

Item 1A.h. Documentation of Mental Status.

Item 1A.h asks you to rate the completeness and timing of nursing documentation of the patient's mental status. Examples of <u>mental status</u> include the patient's orientation to person, place, or things or the patient's ability to remember recent events.

Item 1A.i. Documentation of Pain.

Item 1A.i asks you about the completeness and timeliness of nursing documentation regarding the patient's experience of pain. This may be either obtained from the patient's complaints or from the nurses' observations of the patient's status, but notes should refer to the presence or absence of pain .   In the absence of specific notations of pain, you should not infer from the documentation of another symptom, such as shortness of breath or anxiety, that pain was assessed.

Item 1A.j. Documentation of Nutritional Intake and Diet.

Item 1A.j asks you to rate the completeness and timeliness of nursing documentation regarding the patient's nutritional intake, type of diet, and food preferences and tolerances.

Item 1A.k. Documentation of Bowel and Bladder Function.

Item 1A.k asks you to rate the completeness and timeliness of nursing documentation regarding the patient's bowel and bladder elimination, e.g., frequency, quantity, continence or incontinence, and chronic status. An admission note which mentions nothing about bowel habits or performance other than "No bowel movement during the last 24 hours" should not be rated as excellent because this documentation provides no information about the patient's chronic bowel status. An excellent rating for the initial assessment should include some mention of duration, e.g., patient is chronically constipated or patient was continent prior to admission, as well as a description of the current bowel status, including any new problems.

Item 1A.l. Documentation of Skin Condition.

Item 1A.l asks you to rate the completeness and timeliness of nursing documentation regarding the patient's skin. By <u>skin condition,</u> we mean documentation of skin integrity, moisture, turgor, color, or any breaks in the skin, e.g., decubitus, as well as signs of perfusion such as temperature.

Item 1A.m. Documentation of Out-of-Hospital Living Arrangements.

Item 1A.m asks you to rate the completeness of nursing documentation regarding the patient's living arrangements outside the hospital. An example of this type of documentation would be the patient's residence prior to admission, such as home or nursing home. This item is rated twice: upon initial assessment and upon preparation for discharge.

Item 1A.n. Documentation of Family/Significant Other Involvement with the Patient.

Item 1A.n asks you to rate the completeness of nursing documentation of observations of family or significant others accompanying the patient at admission, persons who may be involved in decision-making about the patient's care, and/or persons to notify in the event of an emergency, or of the unavailability of such individuals. When rating reassessment, consider the documentation of the person's social contacts, e.g., visits and telephone calls.

QUESTION 1, Part B. General Health Status Assessment for Communicative Patients Only.

If this patient is unable to communicate effectively with nurses (e.g., because of coma, confusion, language or speech barriers), check the box in Column I and skip Part B, proceeding to Part C.

Item 1B.a. Documentation of Psychological State.

Item 1B.a. asks you to rate the completeness and timeliness of nursing documentation regarding the patient's psychological state. By psychological state, we mean description of the patient's mood, such as anxiety or depression.

Item 1B.b. Documentation of Patient's Knowledge of His/Her Condition and Medications.

Item 1B.b asks you to rate the completeness of nursing documentation regarding the patient's knowledge of his/her condition, if the patient is able to communicate. Initial assessment would relate to the patient's reason for being in the hospital, while discharge assessment would relate to his/her understanding of his/her condition and the care required following discharge, including medications

Item 1B.c. Documentation of Orientation to Physical Hospital Environment.

Item 1B.c asks you to rate completeness of nursing documentation of the hospital orientation given to the patient. This item would relate only to the initial assessment. Examples of <u>orientation</u> may be instructions on how to call a nurse, use of the telephone, or visiting hours on the unit or floor.

QUESTION 1, Part C. Diagnosis-Specific Health Status Assessment for Communicative and NonCommunicative Patients.

Item 1C.a. Documentation of Cardiovascular Status.

Item 1C.a asks you to rate the completeness and timeliness of nursing documentation specifically regarding the patient's cardiovascular status. Examples of <u>cardiovascular status</u> assessment may be cardiac rate and rhythm, chest pain, peripheral/dependent edema, and venous distention.

Item 1C.b. Documentation of Respiratory Status.

Item 1C.b asks you to rate the completeness and timeliness of nursing documentation specifically regarding the patient's respiratory status. Examples of <u>respiratory status</u> documentation include rate and rhythm of respiration, breath sounds, and shortness of breath.

QUESTION 2. Physician Orders

Were physician orders which were written on day 1 and day 2 implemented by the nurses exactly as ordered (or more frequently or thoroughly) for vital signs and weight?

Purpose

The purpose of this question is to understand how well the nurses carried out the physicians' orders.

Data Sources

To identify the physicians' orders, use the physicians' order sheets for day 1 and day 2. To assess the nurses' implementation of these orders, use all relevant sections of the medical record (e.g., TPR records, flowsheets, nurses' notes) for the first 5 days of the patient's hospitalization or the length of the hospitalization if the stay was shorter than 5 days.

Rating Scale

Yes: Assign *yes* if the nurses carried out all the physicians' orders from days 1 and 2 exactly as ordered or more frequently or thoroughly.

No: Assign *no* if nurses did not carry out all the physicians' orders from days 1 and 2 or carried them out less frequently or thoroughly than ordered.

SPECIFIC ITEMS

Item a. Vital Signs

Item a asks you to indicate whether the nurses implemented all the physicians' orders from day 1 and day 2 for measuring temperature, pulse, respiration, and blood pressure. In assessing whether the implementation was exactly as ordered, consider completeness, frequency, timing, and any other specifications. As an example, you should assign no if the physician ordered the measurement of vital signs four times a day and they were measured three times a day.

Item b. Weight

Item b asks you to indicate whether the nurses implemented all the physicians' orders from day 1 and day 2 for measuring the patient's weight. In assessing whether the implementation was exactly as ordered, consider completeness, frequency, timing, and any other specifications. Assign no, for example, if a weight was ordered on admission and it was not done, even if the nurses' notes state that weight was not obtained because the patient was too heavy for the scale. If the patient died during the hospitalization, you do not need to consider whether the nurses measured the patient's weight on the day of his or her death.

QUESTION 3. Explicit Identification of Problems

How often did the nurses explicitly identify problems that you would regard as nursing issues for the care of this patient? (To answer this question, think about problems you identified during your review for Question 1 and assess whether nurses actually labeled these problems or listed them in some statement of problems.)

Purpose

The purpose of this question is to understand the extent to which nurses label problems in the medical record. By nursing problems, we mean problems that may affect the health status or outcomes of patients, and that require attention from nurses. By explicitly identify, we mean that the patient's nursing problems are clearly labeled. For example, the patient's nursing problems are stated within a problem list, diagnosis list, care plan, or S.O.A.P. notes. It is not sufficient if problems are mentioned or included in a narrative.

Do not be bothered by the fact that care plans and problem lists were not in frequent use in the early to mid-1980's. We are interested in identifying any records which did have information in this format, not in down-rating records which did not.

Data Sources

Use the data sources for Question 1.

Rating Scale

All or Many Problems Stated: means that you found that nurses explicitly recorded more than 60% of the problems you identified.

About Half of Problems Stated: means that you found that nurses explicitly recorded about 40% to 60% of the problems you identified.

Some Problems Stated: means that you found that nurses explicitly recorded less than 40% of the problems you identified.

No Problems Stated: means that nurses explicitly recorded none of the problems you identified.

QUESTION 4. Need for Nursing Intervention.

Please rate the amount (i.e. quantity and intensity) of nursing intervention needed to provide <u>optimal</u> care for this patient. (To do this, think again about problems you identified during your review of days 1 and 2 for Question 1, and what you would do to manage them.) Focus on what the patient needed; not on what the patient got.

Purpose

The purpose of this question is to assess whether this patient demands a high or low intensity of nursing interventions relative to other CHF patients. A very demanding patient might require multiple interventions for a variety of problems, such as confusion, shortness of breath, anxiety, and high risk for development of pressure ulcers. A very undemanding patient might require only routine monitoring because he or she had only uncomplicated CHF without other chronic illnesses.

Data Sources

Use data sources from Question 1.

Rating Scale

<u>*Above Average Amount of Nursing Interventions*</u>: By above average we mean that this patient needs more nursing interventions than the usual CHF patient.

<u>*About Average Amount of Nursing Interventions*</u>: By about average we mean that this patient needs about the same number of nursing interventions as the usual CHF patient.

<u>*Below Average Amount of Nursing Interventions*</u>: By below average we mean that this patient needs fewer nursing interventions than the usual CHF patient.

QUESTION 5. Nursing Management of Problems

Please rate the quality of nurse management of each specified tracer problem that applies to this patient.

Purpose

This question attempts to determine the quality of the patient's nursing care by examining the management of specific tracer problems.

By <u>tracer problems</u>, we mean common measurable problems whose treatment can be taken as indicative of the overall quality of care. Examples may be diabetes or pulmonary edema in a patient admitted for congestive heart failure. Tracer problems are divided into three categories. Questions 5A1 and 5A2 focus on problems identified during the initial period of hospitalization. 5A.1 lists actual tracer problems, i.e., problems that exist already, based on information from any provider during the days specified in the question. 5A.2 lists actual or potential tracer problems. A potential problem is one that you think the patient is at high risk for having or developing, whether or not the diagnosis has been made by health care providers. You should consider a patient as having an actual or potential problem if they have signs, symptoms, or diagnoses recorded in the record that make the likelihood of having or developing the problem high. 5A.3 asks you to identify changes (worsening) in vital signs during the period after initial hospitalization.

By <u>nursing goals, expected outcomes, or planned actions</u>, we mean a statement of what the nurses hope to achieve with respect to the patient's condition within a certain time frame, or a plan of action that refers to what will be done over time.

By <u>nursing intervention</u>, we mean "any direct care treatment that a nurse performs on behalf of a patient. These treatments include nurse-initiated treatments resulting from nursing diagnosis, physician-initiating treatments resulting from medical diagnoses, and performance of the daily essential functions for the client who cannot do these." (Bulechek and McCloskey, 1989; Bulechek and McCloskey, 1992) Interventions are the actions nurses take to carry through their plans, goals, and expected outcomes, regardless of whether they have specified these plans, goals, and expected outcomes in the medical record.

In asking if the medical record ever indicated whether the nurse recorded or evaluated the patient's tracer problem as <u>improved, worsened, or the same,</u> we are asking whether the nurse reflected on the patient's progress. By evaluation, we mean the process of determining the client's progress toward the attainment of expected outcomes. Evaluation may be indicated by a determination that the problem has been resolved. A problem is judged to be resolved if the patient has attained expected outcomes and requires no further special attention for the problem (although routine assessments continue), e.g., patient now mobile or skin intact or no longer at high risk. The problem is judged to be unresolved if the patient has not attained expected outcomes, e.g., patient remains immobile or still has skin breakdown. An unresolved problem may have remained unchanged, improved somewhat but not completely, or have worsened.

Data Sources

Identify the problems in Column 5A using usual data sources including the nurse's notes and data records, physician's notes, and consults. For 5A.1 and 5A.2, use these sources for the first two days for hospitalization only (days 1,2). To identify changes in status (5A.3), review all vital signs sheets for day 3 and after, and note the date for any new major change in vital signs that was not present on admission. For example, major changes might be a new temperature greater than 101 degrees F or 38 C; new blood pressure level > 180 or > 105 diastolic or < 100 systolic; new heart rate > 130 or < 50; or new high respiratory rate > 30.

After you have identified the problems, assess the nurse's management of these problems in Columns 5B, C, and D based only on nursing records. Begin with the day the problem occurred and review through the subsequent 4 days (total of 5 days).

Rating Scales

5A. For each tracer problem (e.g., fever), you are first asked whether the patient has this problem:

> *No/No Data*: Assign *no/no data* if the patient does not have this problem and proceed to the next problem below in Column 5A (e.g., diabetes). No/no data can mean that the problem was evaluated and determined not to exist or that the problem was not evaluated and/or not commented on.

> *Yes*: Assign *yes* if the patient has this problem and proceed to rate the nursing management of the problem by moving across the page through Columns 5B (nursing plans, goals, and expected outcomes), 5C (nursing interventions) and D (evaluation).

5B. If you assigned *yes* (i.e., if the patient has this problem), you are next asked whether any nursing goals, expected outcomes, or planned actions were specified for this problem in the medical record.

> *Yes*. Assign *yes* if the nurses caring for the patient stated in the medical record at least one nursing care goal, expected outcome, or planned action for this patient. Include goals for problems identified by physicians in notes or orders.

> *No*. Assign *no* if there is no statement of a nursing care goal, expected outcome, or planned action for this problem.

5C. If you assigned *yes* in Column A (i.e., if the patient has this problem), rate whether appropriate nursing interventions were carried out as follows:

> *Yes, all*: Assign this rating if you, as the nurse caring for this patient, would not need to perform any more interventions to optimally manage the problem.

> *Yes, Most:* Assign this rating if you believe that, as the nurse caring for this patient, most of the appropriate nursing interventions were performed but you would need to do a few additional interventions to optimally manage the problem.

> *Yes, Some*: Assign this rating if some of the appropriate nursing interventions were carried out, but as the nurse caring for this

patient, you would need to do considerably more or different interventions to optimally manage the problem.

No, none: Assign this rating if the patient has this problem but you found no evidence at all in the record that appropriate nursing interventions were carried out to manage that problem.

5D. If you assigned *yes* in Column A (i.e., the patient has this problem), you are also asked whether the nurses caring for the patient explicitly stated in the record whether the symptom, sign, or problem improved, worsened, or stayed the same. A statement that a worrisome or positive symptom increased or decreased can be counted, e.g., "shortness of breath increased" or "less redness," but two measurements by themselves should not be counted, e.g., respiration on day 1 = 20 and respiration on day 2 = 30.

Yes. Assign *yes* if you find at least one statement that this problem improved, worsened, or stayed the same.

No. Assign *no* if you find no statement that this problem improved, worsened, or stayed the same.

SPECIFIC ITEMS

QUESTION 5, Part 5A.1: Actual Tracer Problems

Item a. Fever.

Item a asks you to rate the quality of the nursing management of fever. We would define the patient as <u>febrile</u> if the patient's record mentions the word fever or the patient has a temperature greater than 101°F.

Item b. Diabetes.

Item b asks you to rate the quality of the nursing management of diabetes. We define CHF patient as at high risk for <u>diabetes</u> if physicians or nurses have noted diabetes mellitus in the medical record or hyperglycemia >200 based on blood sugar recordings.

Item c. Anxiety or Depression.

Item c asks you to rate the quality of the nursing management of anxiety or depression (affect, mood, behavior) documented by a physician or nurse.

Item d. Self-Care Deficit with Feeding

Item d asks you to rate the quality of the nursing management of a feeding deficit. We define the CHF patient as having a <u>feeding deficit</u> if he or she has an impaired ability to perform eating or swallowing activities.

Item e. Impaired Physical Mobility Including Activity Intolerance.

Item e asks you to rate the quality of the nursing management of impaired physical mobility.   We define the CHF patient as having <u>impaired physical mobility</u> if nurses' or physicians' notes indicate that the patient has difficulty moving including moving in bed, transferring, sitting or ambulating. We define the CHF patient as at high risk for <u>activity intolerance</u> if the patient's record mentions such signs as a complaint of weakness or fatigue, pallor, diaphoresis or shortness of breath on exertion.

Item f. Shock or Blood Pressure < 90 systolic.

Item f asks you to rate the quality of nursing management of shock. We define shock as a mention of the word in the record, or a blood pressure ≤ 90 systolic.

Item g. Chest Pain

Item g asks you to rate the quality of nursing management of chest pain. By <u>chest pain</u>, we mean a notation in the record indicating that the patient experienced chest pain, cardiac pain, or possible or probable cardiac pain.

Item h. Non-Cardiac Pain.

Item h asks you to rate the quality of nursing management of pain other than chest pain or pain that has been identified by health care providers as likely to be cardiac. Shortness of breath should not be included.

Item i. Knowledge Deficit Regarding His/Her Condition and Medications.

Item i asks you to rate the quality of nursing management of the patient's educational needs regarding his or her medical condition and medications. Since all patients require some education about their condition and medication, circle 1 in Column 5A for all communicative patients (indicating the patient does have the problem.) If patient is non-communicative, this item does not apply and 9 should be circled.

QUESTION 5, Part 5A.2: Actual or Potential Tracer Problems

Item a. Pulmonary Edema/Pulmonary Congestion.

Item a asks you to rate the quality of the nursing management of actual or potential pulmonary edema/pulmonary congestion. We define the congestive heart failure (CHF) patient as having probable or actual <u>pulmonary edema or pulmonary congestion</u> if he or she has shortness of breath, pulse > 130, respiratory rate > 30, or cyanosis documented in physicians or nurses notes.

Item b. Actual or High Risk for Impaired Skin Integrity.

Item b asks you to rate the quality of the management of actual or potential impaired skin integrity. We define the CHF patient as at high risk for <u>impaired skin integrity</u> if the patient's medical record mentions pedal or sacral edema, coma, decubitus, incontinence, limited bed or chair mobility, or poor nutrition. We realize that most elderly CHF patients are at risk for pressure ulcers; however, in this question we are interested only in those who are at high risk. In 5C, consider interventions directed at the risk factors as well as impaired skin integrity.

Item c. Dysrhythmias.

Item c asks you to rate the quality of the nursing management of actual or potential dysrhythmias. We would define the CHF patient as at high risk for <u>dysrhythmias</u> if he or she has irregular pulse, heart beat, or arrhythmia on cardiac monitor documented in physician or nurse's notes. You may identify this problem based on EKG results with a formal interpretation that nurses could have read or a notation in the physicians' progress notes, but not based on uninterpreted EKGs.

Item d. High Risk for Injury Secondary to Confusion.

Item d asks you to rate the quality of the nursing management of actual or potential injury secondary to confusion. We define the CHF patient as at high risk for <u>in-hospital injury</u> if the patient's medical record mentions that the patient is confused, disoriented, or somnolent.

Item e. Other.

Item e asks you to rate the quality of the nursing management of the one other problem, if any, you consider most essential for the patient's care. Please specify the problem.

QUESTION 5, Part 5A.3: Change in Status

Item a. Change in Vital Signs

Item a asks you to rate the quality of the nursing management of changes in vital signs that occur after day 2 of admission. By change in vital signs, we mean new onset of a fever (T > 101° F), hypotension (systolic ≤ 100), severe hypertension (systolic > 180 or diastolic > 105), tachypnea (respiratory rate > 30), tachycardia (rate > 130) or bradycardia (rate < 50) that were _not_ present on admission (days 1 and 2). Use only vital signs flowsheets. For this question, ignore vital signs recorded in narrative nurses' notes or other records. Limit your review to vital signs flowsheets from day 3 and after.

QUESTION 6. Appropriateness of Nursing Interventions

Whether or not all the problems you detected as you reviewed the medical record were explicitly recorded by nurses, rate the degree to which the nurses <u>carried out</u> the appropriate interventions for all these problems (including changing the frequency of monitoring).

Purpose

The purpose of this question is to estimate the degree to which problems that you would have identified based on the assessment data recorded were recognized by these nurses as problems and led to appropriate nursing interventions, regardless of whether the problems were explicitly recorded in problem lists in the medical record. By nursing <u>problems,</u> we mean problems that may affect the health status or outcomes of patients, and that require attention from nurses.. The assessment data provide the basis upon which patient problems are identified. By nursing <u>interventions</u>, we mean any direct care treatments that a nurse performs on behalf of a patient. These treatments include nurse-initiated treatments and performance of daily essential functions for the patient who cannot do these for him/herself. For example, the nurse's administration of an antipyretic and cooling measure follows logically from assessment data indicating a fever.

You may frequently find that nurses did not explicitly identify problems (or record nursing care plans in the medical record), yet performed timely intervention for all problems you could identify based on the clinical data.

Data Sources

Use data sources for Questions 1 and 4 above.

Rating Scale

All or Most Carried Out: means that you found that nurses carried out about 60% or more of the appropriate interventions.

About Half Carried Out: means that you found that nurses carried out about 50% of appropriate interventions.

Some Carried Out: means that you found that nurses carried out about 20% to 40 % of the interventions.

Few or None Carried Out: Few or none of the appropriate interventions were carried out (e.g., fewer than 20% carried out).

QUESTION 7. Quality of Medication Administration Documentation

What is the quality of nurses' documentation related to medication administration and actual or potential medication side effects?

Purpose

The purpose of Question 6 is to assess the completeness of the nurse's record keeping on the identification of the medications administered to the patient, the time and amounts of their administration, and any side effects or potential side effects of medications administered during the hospital stay. The record should show that the nurses were attentive to the possibility of side effects.

Data Sources

The data sources for this question are medication records and nurses' notes.

Rating Scale

Excellent: Assign *excellent* if the documentation would provide you, as a registered nurse newly assigned to care for this patient, all the information you would need to know about the administration of inhospital medications to continue to safely and accurately administer medications.

Good:: Assign *good* if the documentation would provide you, as a registered nurse newly assigned to care for this patient, most of the information you would need to know about the administration of inhospital medications to continue to safely and accurately administer medications.

Fair:: Assign *fair* if the documentation would provide you, as a registered nurse newly assigned to care for this patient, some of the information you would need to know about the administration of inhospital medications to continue to safely and accurately administer medications.

Poor: Assign *poor* if the documentation would provide you, as the registered nurse newly assigned to care for this patient, little of the information you would need to know about the administration of inhospital medications to continue to safely and accurately administer medications.

QUESTION 8. Adverse Nursing Events

Did any of the specified adverse nursing events occur during this hospitalization?

Purpose

The purpose of question 6 is to determine whether the patient experienced any of the specified negative events during his/her course of hospitalization.

Data Sources

The data sources for this question include the nursing records, medication sheets, and any special reports for days 1 through 10, if applicable, and the day of and day prior to discharge.

Rating Scale

Yes: Assign *yes* if at least one such event occurred.

No/No Data: Assign *no/no data* if there is no evidence that such an event occurred.

SPECIFIC ITEMS

Item 8.a. Medication Error.

Item 8.a asks you to indicate whether any medication errors were evident. Please count a <u>medication</u> as being given in <u>error</u> only if the wrong medication was given or if the wrong dose was given.

Item 8.b. Fall.

Item 8.b asks you to indicate whether the patient fell. during the hospitalization, regardless of whether or not the patient sustained fractures or injury. By <u>fall</u>, we mean that the patient's position unintentionally and abruptly changed from a bed, chair, or standing position to a lowered position such as the floor.

Item 8.c. Underdosing of a PRN Medication.

Item 8.c asks whether there is evidence of an underdose of PRN medication. By underdosing, we mean that a medication was not given, an appropriate amount was not given, or the medication was not given frequently enough to relieve the symptom. For example, an underdose of pain medication would be indicated if the medication administered for pain was a smaller dose than that allowable and yet there was a notation that the patient was experiencing pain within two hours of the administration, while the expected duration of action was 4 hours.

Item 8.d. Overdosing of PRN Medication.

Item 8.d asks whether there is evidence of an overdose of a PRN medication. By overdosing, we mean that the amount or frequency was such that the patient could have been harmed. For example, an overdose of PRN medication would be indicated if the nurse continued to administer one or more additional doses after adverse effect or a longer period of effect than expected was evident.

Item 8.e. Patient Discharged Unstable.

Item 8.e asks whether the patient was discharged in an unstable condition, i.e., with problems that you think should have been corrected before discharge and that are likely to cause poor outcomes if not corrected. Circle 9 if the patient died in the hospital.

Item 8.f. Other. Specify.

Item 8.f asks whether one or more adverse effects other than the ones listed occurred. Include cases in which medication use may have reflected poor judgment but was not overtly an overdose or underdose. Also include instances where nursing action showed poor judgment which could have resulted in poor outcomes. Please specify what these adverse events were.

8A. Reviewer Instructions

If you answered *Yes* to any item (a-f) in Question 8, i.e., at least one of these adverse nursing events occurred during the care of this patient, answer Question 9.

If you answered *No/No data* to every item (a-f) in Question 8, i.e., there was no evidence that any of these events occurred, skip to Question 10.

QUESTION 9. Adverse Event Management

If there were adverse nursing events, rate how well the nurse managed the problem. (If there were more than one problem, rate the first one on the list).

Purpose

The purpose of question 9 is to assess the appropriateness of the nurse's intervention in response to negative events. For example, if the patient fell, were appropriate measures taken with respect to the fall? Interventions may range from handling the immediate event to managing the acute symptoms to actions designed to prevent similar adverse events in the future. In the case of falls, you might consider the most important interventions would be those directed towards prevention. On the other hand, the most important interventions in a patient with respiratory depression due to pain medication overdose might be directed toward rapidly improving respiratory status.

Data Source

Use the same data sources as for Question 8.

Rating Scale

Extremely Well: Assign this rating if the management of the event matched the ideal of how you think the adverse event should have been managed.

Well: Assign *well* if you think the management of the adverse event was above average, although not ideal.

Adequately: Assign *adequately* if you think the management of the adverse event would be considered acceptable.

Poorly: Assign *poorly* if the management of the adverse event was such that additional measures would have been needed to ensure an acceptable outcome.

Very Poorly: Assign *very poorly* if the management of the adverse event was likely to lead to unacceptable outcomes.

QUESTION 10. Need for Nursing Time

How much nursing time would it take to provide optimal care to the patient described in this medical record, compared to most CHF patients?

Purpose

The purpose of this question is to evaluate how time consuming optimal nursing care to this patient would be relative to other CHF patients. By optimal care, we mean care that maximizes the probability of good outcomes. Think in terms of the care needed, not in terms of the care actually received by the patient.

Data Source:

The data sources include the nursing records, medication sheets, and special reports for day 1 through 10, if applicable, and the day of and day prior to discharge.

Rating Scale

More Than Average Time: Assign if you think that it would take more nursing time to provide optimal care to this patient than to most other CHF patients.

Average Time: Assign *average time* if you think that it would take about the same amount of nursing time to provide optimal care to this patient as to most other CHF patients.

Less Than Average Time: Assign *less than average time* if you think it would take less nursing time to provide optimal care to this patient than to most CHF patients.

QUESTION 11. Need for Nursing Expertise

How much nursing expertise would it take to provide optimal care to the patient described in this medical record, compared to most CHF patients?

Purpose

The purpose of this question is to assess the amount of nursing expertise you judge to be necessary to provide optimal care to this patient relative to most other CHF patients. By optimal care, we mean care that maximizes the probability of good outcomes.

Data Source

Use the same data sources as for Question 10.

Rating Scale

More Than Average Expertise: Assign *more than average expertise* if you think that it would take more nursing expertise to provide optimal care to this patient than to most other CHF patients.

Average Expertise: Assign *average expertise* if you think that it would take about the same amount of nursing expertise, to provide optimal care to this patient as to most CHF patients.

Less Than Average Expertise: Assign *less than average expertise* you think that it would take less nursing expertise to provide optimal care to this patient than to most other CHF patients.

QUESTION 12. Need for Nursing Special Training

How much could this patient benefit from care by a nurse with special training in geriatrics or cardiology, compared to care by nurses without this special training?

Purpose

The purpose of this question is to assess whether or not specialized training, knowledge, or skills in geriatric or cardiac care would benefit this patient.

Data Source

Use the same data sources as for Question 10.

Rating Scale

Benefit Greatly: Use this rating if a nurse with special training would be very likely to have a significant impact on the patient's health outcomes.

Benefit Somewhat: Use this rating if a nurse with special training is somewhat likely to have a significant impact on the patient's health outcomes.

Little or No Benefit : Use this rating if a nurse with special training is unlikely to have a significant impact on the patient's health outcomes.

QUESTION 13. Patient Discharge

Answer 13A if the patient was discharged alive.

Answer 13B if the patient died during this hospitalization.

QUESTION 13A.

PATIENT DISCHARGED ALIVE: How would you characterize this patient's condition at discharge, <u>given this patient's status at admission</u> (hospital days 1 and 2)?

Purpose

The purpose of this question is to evaluate how you would describe this patient's condition at discharge in comparison to what you would expect, given his or her health status at admission and the evaluation of tracer problems during hospitalization.

Data Source

The data source would include the patient's complete medical record from days 1 and 2 of admission (to assess expectations) and the day of and day prior to discharge (to assess the patient's status at discharge).

Rating Scale

<u>Much better than expected</u>: Assign *much better than expected* if the patient's condition at discharge was far beyond what you might have expected given his or her health status at admission and the evaluation of tracer problems during hospitalization.

<u>Better than expected</u>: Assign *better than expected* if the patient's condition at discharge was somewhat better than you would have expected given his or her status at admission and the evaluation of tracer problems during hospitalization.

<u>As expected</u>: Assign *as expected* if the patient's condition at discharge was what you would have expected, given his or her health status at admission and the evaluation of tracer problems during hospitalization.

Worse than expected: Assign *worse than expected* if the patient's condition at discharge was somewhat worse than you would have expected, given his or her health status at admission and the evaluation of tracer problems during hospitalization.

Much worse than expected: Assign *much worse than expected* if the patient's condition at discharge was far worse than you might have expected given his or her health status at admission and the evaluation of tracer problems during hospitalization.

QUESTION 13B.

PATIENT WAS DISCHARGED DEAD: How would you characterize the death, <u>given this patient's status at admission</u> (hospital days 1 and 2)?

Purpose

The purpose of this question is to evaluate how you would describe this person's death in comparison to what you would expect, given his or her health status at admission would lead you to expect.

Data Source

The data source would include the patient's complete medical record from days 1 and 2 of hospitalization.

Rating Scale

<u>*Definitely expected*</u>: Assign *definitely expected* if the person's death was clearly what you expected given his or her health status at admission.

<u>*Somewhat expected*</u>: Assign *somewhat expected* if the person's death was not clearly expected given his or her health status at admission, but was not surprising either.

<u>*Somewhat unexpected*</u>: Assign *somewhat unexpected* if you were somewhat surprised that the patient died given his or her health status at admission.

<u>*Definitely unexpected*</u>: Assign *definitely unexpected* if you would have clearly expected the person to live, based on his or her health status at admission.

QUESTION 14. Quality of Patient Services

How would you characterize the quality of the specified services delivered to this patient?

Purpose

The purpose of this question is to assess the overall quality of the nursing and physician services from a nursing perspective.

Data Source

Use all relevant parts of the medical record such as nursing records, physician's history, examination and progress reports, lab reports, flow sheet, physiotherapy notes, or records of other services.

Rating Scale

<u>Excellent</u>: Assign *excellent* if the quality of the care and the use of services matched your idea of how this care should have been provided for the optimal benefit of the patient.

<u>Good</u>: Assign *good* if the quality of the care provided or the use of services approximated but did not exactly match your ideal of how this care should have been provided for the optimal benefit of the patient.

<u>Fair</u>: Assign *fair* if the quality of the care provided or the use of services were less than ideal and there would have been some chance that harm resulted.

<u>Poor</u>: Assign *poor* if the quality of the care provided or the use of services fell far short of ideal and if it is likely that some patients treated in this way would have worse than expected outcomes.

SPECIFIC ITEMS

Item 14.a. Nursing Care.

Item 14.a asks you to rate the overall quality of nursing care, including assessments, interventions, and evaluations.

Item 14.b. Physician Care.

Item 14.b asks you to rate the overall quality of physician care. From a nursing perspective, did the physician care seem sensible and responsive? For example, if a nurse's note indicates the patient was restless or agitated, was there evidence that soon thereafter the physician evaluated the patient or wrote a new set of orders that were appropriate to the patient's restlessness or agitation.

QUESTION 15. Overall Quality of Care

Considering everything you know about this patient, please rate overall quality of care.

Purpose
This question asks you to specify your overall assessment of the care delivered to this patient.

Data Source
Use all relevant information in the medical record to address this question.

Rating Scale
Extreme, Above Standard : Assign *extreme, above standard* if you feel the overall care delivered was ideal.

Above Standard: Assign *above standard* if you feel there are some aspects of care missing, but it was still above average.

Adequate: Assign *adequate* if you feel that the care was average.

Below Standard: Assign *below standard* if you feel the care given had some acceptable aspects but was below average overall.

Extreme, Below Standard: Assign *extreme, below standard* if you feel the care delivered was almost completely unacceptable.

QUESTION 16. Rating of Nurses

Would you want your mother cared for by these <u>nurses</u> in this hospital?

Purpose

This question is designed to integrate your thought and judgment with your feelings and intuition regarding the nursing care provided.

Data Source

Use all relevant information in the medical record.

Rating Scale

Definitely Yes: Assign *definitely yes* if overall you judge the nursing care given to far exceed acceptable.

Probably Yes: Assign *probably yes* if overall you judge the care given to be acceptable.

Probably No: Assign *probably no* if you have the feeling that there is something amiss in the nursing care provided.

Definitely No: Assign *definitely no* if the nursing care delivered feels unacceptable.

QUESTION 17. Rating of Physicians

Would you want your mother cared for by these <u>physicians </u>in this hospital?

Purpose

This question is designed to integrate your thought and judgment with your feelings and intuition regarding the physician care provided.

Data Source

Use all relevant information in the medical record.

Rating Scale

<u>*Definitely Yes*</u>: Assign *definitely yes* if overall you judge the medical care given to far exceed acceptable.

<u>*Probably Yes*</u>: Assign *probably yes* if overall you judge the medical care given to be acceptable.

<u>*Probably No*</u>: Assign *probably no* if you have the feeling that there is something amiss in the medical care provided.

<u>*Definitely No*</u>: Assign *definitely no* if the medical care delivered feels unacceptable.

QUESTION 18. Charting Methods

Possible methods of charting are specified.

QUESTION 18A.

Which of the following charting methods were used in this medical record?

QUESTION 18B.

Of the methods circled in Question 18A, which one method was used the most to record information about the type and course of the patient's nursing problems or diagnoses and interventions?

Purpose

The purpose of this question is to determine the various types of documentation that were used by nurses for this patient during his or her hospitalization. We are interested in understanding the extent to which the type of recording in the medical record affects ratings of nursing care.

Data Source

Use all nurses' charting in the medical record to answer these questions.

Rating Scale

In Question 18A, circle the number of each method that was used. More than one method may be circled.

In Question 18B, enter the number of the *one* method which was used the most to record information about the type and course of the patient's nursing problems or diagnoses and interventions. Only one number may be entered.

SPECIFIC ITEMS

Nurses' Notes (without problem focus).

This item asks you whether nurses' notes were used in this medical record. By <u>nurses' notes</u>, we mean handwritten, descriptive accounts by the nurse, which predominately include assessment data and interventions performed. These notes are structured by chronological order or aspects of care. Within these descriptive notes, there may be evidence of a patient care problem, but the notes are not organized by problem.

Problem Oriented Method of Recording (POMR)

This item asks you whether POMR is used in the documentation. By <u>POMR</u>, we mean a structured form of handwritten charting, which is organized by problem focus. Problems or diagnoses are numbered and listed. This form of charting may use a SOAP or SOAPIE format. SOAP = Subjective, Objective, Analysis, Plan. SOAPIE = Subjective, Objective, Analysis, Plans, Intervention, Evaluation.

Preprinted Nursing Care Plans, e.g., Standard Care Plans.

This item asks you whether preprinted nursing care plans are used in the documentation. By <u>preprinted nursing care plans,</u> we mean sheets prepared in advance of the patient's admission that are commonly considered "standard care plans," usually with some space provided for the nurse to indicate in handwriting the individualization of the plan of care for the specific patient.

On-line Computerized Forms (excluding nursing care plans), e.g., Computerized Medication Forms.

This item asks you whether on-line computerized forms are used for documentation. By <u>on-line computerized forms,</u> we mean charting on flow charts for physiological monitoring or medication sheets which are printed out by a computerized system. These types of forms can be distinguished (from hand augmented non-computerized preprinted forms) by the automatic entry of timing of events and presence of computerized tracking notations. All or nearly all of the entries will appear to be computer generated/printed; there usually will not be any handwritten additions to this form.

On-line Computerized Nursing Care Plans.

This item asks you whether computerized nursing care plans are used in the documentation. By <u>computerized nursing care plans</u>, we mean nurses' notes which contain nursing care plans including: statements of nursing diagnoses, expected outcomes, interventions, and actual outcomes and/or problem resolution. This type of record can be distinguished by the automatic entry of timing of events and presence of computerized tracking notations. All of these nurse's entries will have been selected at a terminal and printed; therefore, the records usually will not have handwritten additions.

Charting by Exception.

This item asks you whether charting by exception is used in the documentation. By <u>charting by exception</u>, we mean a method of charting where the nurse is responsible for recording an initial patient assessment. Subsequent data are recorded only if a) they are positive findings (e.g., calf pain with positive Homan's sign) or b) there is a change in the initial assessment data recorded. Less than 20% of the chart will be accounted for by comments that particular findings are normal or unchanged.

Other.

This item asks you whether any other method of charting is used in the documentation. By <u>other</u> methods, we mean any other recognizable type of charting which could affect the quality of care. If more than one other method is used, specify the one which you think most affects patient care.

QUESTION 19. Additional Forms

In addition to medication, IV, TPR, ICU, and intake and output flowsheet records, which of the specified forms were present in the record?

Purpose

The purpose of this question is to determine whether forms other than the universal medication sheet, TPR , ICU, and intake and output sheets were present in the record. Again, we are interested in understanding the extent to which the type of recording in the medical record affects ratings of nursing care. Count a form if it is present, even if it is not used.

To be counted, #1,2, or 3 should be a separate sheet in the chart and should contain at least three domains of care or multiple categories within one domain. Examples of <u>domains</u> may be activities of daily living, functional status, or neurological assessment. Examples of <u>categories</u> within the domain of pressure ulcers are skin color, size of lesion, depth of lesion, and treatment provided. The sheet should contain a space either for a check or for a brief notation next to the domain or category printed on the form.

For #4, by <u>Kardex or care plan sheet</u>, we mean a form with columns for problem list, interventions, and dates.

Data Source

Use nursing documentation other than narrative nurses' notes and progress records to address this question.

Rating Scale

Circle the number if the checklist or flowsheet was used. Leave the space blank if it was not used. More than one checklist or flowsheet may be circled.

SPECIFIC ITEMS

Activity, Functional Status, or Neurological Record.

This item asks you whether an activity record checklist, functional status checklist, or neurological checklist was found in the medical record. By activity record checklist, we mean a form on which nurses may indicate the amount of time the patient was sitting up in a chair or ambulating, as well as how well the patient tolerated the activity. This form may have spaces provided for the nurse to write in the date and time and check the indicated activity for the patient. By functional status checklist, we mean a form which allows the nurse to place a check mark to indicate the level of the patient's ability to perform activities of daily living such as the ability to feed, dress, and bathe self. By neurological status checklist, we mean a form which allows the nurse to place a check mark to indicate the level of consciousness and/or change in motor or sensory ability. A standardized scale is often pre-printed for this purpose and, once completed, becomes part of the patient's medical record.

Disease or Condition Oriented Sheet (e.g., Diabetes or Pressure Ulcer Record.

This item asks you whether a disease or condition oriented record, such as a diabetic record or pressure ulcer record was found in the medical record. A diabetic record or checklist is a form which allows the nurse to place a check mark to indicate the administration of antidiabetic agents and record the value of blood glucose testing and other activities related to direct diabetic care of the patient. As another example, a pressure ulcer or decubitus care flowsheet is a form which allows the nurse to indicate (by checkmarks, numbers, or brief description) the location, size, and extent of the pressure ulcers and the treatment administered on designated dates and times.

Other Specialized Sheet (e.g., Teaching Record).

This item asks you whether another kind of specialized sheet, such as a patient/family teaching record, was found in the medical record. By the example of a patient/family teaching record, we mean a form which allows the nurse to briefly describe or place a check mark to indicate the extent to which various aspects of care have been taught to the patient and/or family.

Form Resembling Patient Kardex or Care Plan Sheet (e.g., Form with Columns for Problem List, Interventions, and Dates).

This item asks you whether a Kardex, care plan sheet, or other form with columns for problem list, interventions, and dates was found in the medical record.

COMMENTS:

Space is provided for any comments you wish to give us regarding your review of this medical record.

REMINDER:

When you have completed the implicit review, please carefully review each page of the form to insure that all questions are answered.

REFERENCES

Burrell LO. *Adult Nursing in Hospital and Community Settings.* Norwalk, CN:Appleton & Lange, 1992.

Carnevali DL, Mitchell PH, Woods NF, Tanner CA. *Diagnostic Reasoning in Nursing.* Philadelphia, PA:Lippincott, 1984.

Carpenito LJ. *Nursing Care Plans and Documentation.* Philadelphia, PA:Lippincott, 1991.

Carpenito LJ. *Nursing Diagnosis.* (5th Edition.) Philadelphia, PA:Lippincott. 1993.

Draper D, Kahn KL, Reinisch EJ, Sherwood MJ, Carney MF, Kosecoff J, et al. Studying the effects of the DRG-based prospective payment system on quality of care: Design, sampling, and fieldwork. *The Journal of the American Medical Association.* 1990;264:1956-1961.

Gordon M. *Nursing Diagnosis: Process and Application.* (3rd Edition.) St. Louis, MO:Mosby-Year Book, Inc., 1994.

Johnson M, Maas M. Nurse-focused patient outcomes: Challenge for the nineties. In McClosky J and Grace HK (eds), *Current Issues in Nursing.* (4th Edition.) St. Louis, MO:Mosby-Year Book, Inc., 1994.

Kahn KL, Draper D, Keeler EB, Rogers WH, Rubenstein LV, Kosecoff J, et al. *The Effects of the DRG-Based Prospective Payment System on Quality of Care for Hospitalized Medicare Patients: Final Report.* Santa Monica, CA: The RAND Corporation. R-3931-HCFA, 1992.

Kahn KL, Rogers WH, Rubenstein LV, Sherwood MJ, Reinisch EJ, Keeler EB, et al. Measuring quality of care with explicit process criteria pre- and post-implementation of the DRG-based prospective

payment system. *The Journal of the American Medical Association.*
1990b;264:1969-1973.

Kahn KL, Rubenstein LV, Draper D, Kosecoff J, Rogers WH, Keeler EB,
et al. The effects of the DRG-based prospective payment system on
quality care for hospitalized Medicare patients: An introduction
to the series. *The Journal of the American Medical Association.*
1990a;264:1953-1955.

Kahn KL, Rubenstein LV, Sherwood MJ, Brook RH. *Structured Implicit
Review for Physician Implicit Measurement of Quality of Care:
Development of the Form and Guidelines for Its Use.* Santa Monica,
CA:RAND. N-3016-HCFA, 1989.

Lang NM, Clinton JF. Assessment of quality of nursing care. In
Werley HH and Fitzpatric JJ (eds), *Annual Review of Nursing
Research: Vol. 2.* New York, NY:Springer, 1984.

Lang NM, Kraegel JM, Rantz MJ, Krejci JW. *Quality of Health Care for
Older People in America: A Review of Nursing Studies.* Kansas
City, MO:American Nurses Association, 1990.

Lyons TF, Payne BC. The relationship of physicians' medical
recording performance to their medical care performance. *Medical
Care.* 1974;12(5):463-470.

McCormick KA. Future data needs for quality of care monitoring, DRG
considerations, reimbursement and outcome measurement. *IMAGE:
Journal of Nursing Scholarship.* 1991;23(1):29-32.

Moorehead MA, Donaldson RS, Seravalli MR. Comparisons between OEO
Neighborhood Health Centers and other health care providers of
ratings of the quality of health care. *American Journal of Public
Health.* 1971;16(7):1294-1305.

National Center for Nursing Research. *Patient Outcomes Research:
Examining the Effectiveness of Nursing Practice, Proceedings of the
State of the Science Conference* sponsored by the National Center

for Nursing Research, September 11-13, 1991. Washington, DC:National Institutes of Health, NIH Publication No. 93-3411, October 1992.

Rantz MJ. *Nursing Quality Measurement: A Review of Nursing Studies.* Washington, DC:American Nurses Association, 1995.

Richardson FM. Peer review of medical care. *Medical Care.* 1972;10(1):29-39.

Rubenstein LV, Kahn KL, Reinisch EJ, Sherwood MJ, Rogers WH, Brook RH. *Structured Implicit Review of the Medical Record: A Method for Measuring the Quality of In-hospital Medical Care, and a Summary of Quality Changes Following Implementation of Medicare Prospective Payment System.* Santa Monica, CA:RAND. N-3033-HCFA, 1991.

Rubenstein LV, Kahn KL, Reinisch EJ, Sherwood MJ, Rogers WH, Brook RH. Structured implicit review of the medical record: A new method of quality assessment. *Clinical Research.* 1989;37:324A.

Rubenstein LV, Kahn KL, Reinisch EJ, Sherwood MJ, Rogers WH, Kamberg C, et al. Changes in quality of care for five diseases measured by implicit review, 1981 to 1986. *The Journal of the American Medical Association.* 1990;264:1974-1979.

Rubenstein LV, Mates S, Sidel VW. Quality of care assessment by process and outcome scoring. *Annals of Internal Medicine.* 1977;86:617-625.

Rubin HR, Kahn KL, Rubenstein LV, Sherwood MJ. *Guidelines For Structured Implicit Review of the Quality of Hospital Care for Diverse Medical and Surgical Conditions.* Santa Monica, CA:RAND. N-3066-HCFA, 1990.

Rubin HR, Rogers WH, Kahn KL, Rubenstein LV, Brook RH. Watching the doctor-watchers: How well do peer review organization methods detect hospital care quality problems? *The Journal of the American Medical Association.* 1992;267:2349-2354.

Thompson JM, McFarland GK, Hirsch JE, Tucker SM. *Clinical Nursing.* (3rd Edition.) St. Louis, MO:Mosby-Year Book, Inc., 1993.